Private Practice in Occupational Therapy

The *Occupational Therapy in Health Care* series,
Florence S. Cromwell, Editor

Private Practice in Occupational Therapy

Florence S. Cromwell
Editor

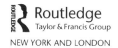

Routledge
Taylor & Francis Group

NEW YORK AND LONDON

First Published by

The Haworth Press, Inc., 28 East 22 Street, New York, NY 10010

This edition published 2011 by Routledge
711 Third Avenue, New York, NY 10017
2 Park Square, Milton Park, Abingdon, Oxon, OX14 4RN

Private Practice in Occupational Therapy has also been published as *Occupational Therapy in Health Care,* Volume 2, Number 2, Summer 1985.

Library of Congress Cataloging in Publication Data
Main entry under title:

Private practice in occupational therapy.

   "Has also been published as Occupational therapy in health care, volume 2, number 2, summer 1985"—T.p. verso.
   Includes bibliographies and index.
   1. Occupational therapy—Practice.
I. Cromwell, Florence S. [DNLM: 1. Occupational Therapy. 2. Private Practice. W1 0C601H v.2 no. 2 / WB 555 P961]
RM735.4.P75 1985   615.8'5152'068   85-5513
ISBN 0-86656-411-X
ISBN 0-86656-412-8 (pbk.)

Publisher's Note
The publisher has gone to great lengths to ensure the quality of this reprint
but points out that some imperfections in the original may be apparent.

Private Practice in Occupational Therapy

Occupational Therapy in Health Care
Volume 2, Number 2

CONTENTS

DIANE SHAPIRO, MA, OTR, *Director Therapeutic Activities, Department of Psychiatry-Westchester Division, The New York Hospital-Cornell Medical Center, White Plains, NY*

SUSAN L. SMITH, MA, LOTR, FAOTA, *Director, Professional Occupational Therapy Services, Metairie, LA*

LYLA M. SPELBRING, PhD, OTR, FAOTA, *Former Head of Department of Associated Health Professions, Eastern Michigan University, Ypsilanti*

JANET C. STONE, BA, OTR, *Former Department Head, Occupational Therapy, Rancho Los Amigos Hospital, Downey, California, and Initiating Editor, AOTA Bulletin on Practice, Huntington Beach, CA*

CARL SUNDSTROM, MA, OTR, LTC, AMSC, *Occupational Therapy Staff Officer, Health Services Command, Fort Sam Houston, TX*

ELLEN DUNLEAVEY TAIRA, MPH, OTR, *Consultant in Program Development in Long Term Care and Editor,* Occupational and Physical Therapy in Geriatrics, *Kailua, HI*

JENNIFER WAMBOLDT, OTR/L, *Assistant Director, Occupational Therapy, Schwab Rehabilitation Center, Chicago, IL*

MARY GRACE WASHBURN, MHA, OTR, FAOTA, *Marketing Director, Health Care Design Services, Kirkham, Michael and Associates, Architects, Engineers, and Planners, Denver, Colorado*

CARLOTTA WELLES, MA, OTR, FAOTA, *Consultant, Professional Liability, and Former Chairman, Occupational Therapy Department, Los Angeles City College, Los Angeles, CA*

Private Practice in
Occupational Therapy

FROM THE EDITOR'S DESK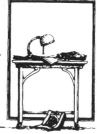

One of the fastest growing segments of occupational therapy practice is in the private practice arena where therapists, alone or in teams of colleagues, are venturing into the market place to offer a tantalizing assortment of needed health care services. According to some of the writers in this issue, "it is about time!"

In putting together the issue it was difficult to plan and select papers that would provide you, the reader, with both the diversity and the excitement represented in the models of practice now found in our profession. The issue is a large one, and could have been larger. Despite its scope, many of you will wish we had included such things as school system consultation, hand practices, well-child developmental programs, consultation to architects and community planners, and stories of the specialists who are vendors of various assistive equipment. Perhaps another issue later can address those roles and others that are only now emerging in private practice.

Your attention however is drawn to some models of entrepreneurism already reported in previous issues of *OTHC:* Vol. I-2, Tooper as an itinerant educator and purveyor of special strategies for treatment and management uses . . . humor; Vol. I-4, Fink who is an expert designer and engineer of adaptive equipment; Vol. II-1, Grover who developed a "brokerage" for services to/for the aged and their families.

Occupational therapists can indeed be innovators and risk takers in addressing needs of patients and their communities . . . which brings us to the message of our PRACTICE WATCH feature in this issue by McFadden and Hanschu. It seemed especially fitted as an accompaniment to this theme, as certainly no one in private practice is a stranger to risk taking.

The writers who follow suggest both general and specific ideas and philosophies to guide anyone considering private practice. Frazian offers an especially colorful picture of the climate in which the profession must examine its options and directions for the decade ahead. She strongly suggests the need for entrepreneurship.

Others offer, some in a very personal way, provocative models for private practice, both of direct and indirect services, and an elaboration of the range of elements one must address in a business venture such as a free-standing "clinic". It is not suggested that the collection of papers provides "all you need to know" if you contemplate a business venture of your own. Yet it is hoped you will come away with clearer ideas of the risks, the potentials, and yes, the excitement of this occupational therapy role of independence.

Looking ahead to themes to come in *OTHC* you can anticipate, still this year, an examination of how occupational therapists approach the problems that *adolescence* brings to young persons already suffering from severely disabling conditions. In one issue we shall look at the dynamics of growing into adulthood with spinal cord injury, head trauma, unplanned motherhood, cerebral palsy, arthritis, various kinds and severity of psychiatric illnesses, anorexia, substance abuse and so on. Occupational therapists have special things to offer persons in this age group.

Our final theme in the volume will address more completely the growing practice demand—*work-related programming* in all kinds of settings with patients with many kinds of problems and needs.

On the other hand, we still seek your interest as writers for themes to come . . . all featuring occupational therapy programming with special populations and settings: the *energy-deficient patient* (SCI, cardiac, COPD, frail aged, etc.); *patients with feeding needs* that occupational therapists address; *computer applications* in the profession . . . education, research and practice; and finally how we address the *cultural implications of treatment planning*.

Finally, we thank you for your continued interest and seek your comments and suggestions.

Florence S. Cromwell, Editor

PRACTICE WATCH:
THINGS TO THINK ABOUT

Risk Taking in Occupational Therapy

Susan M. McFadden, MEd, OTR, FAOTA
Bonnie Hanschu, BS, OTR

The word "risk" comes to the English language in the mid-seventeenth century from France as the word "risque". Before the word "risk" existed, the word "hazard" appears to have had the closest meaning as in Shakespeare's *Merchant of Venice:*

Men that hazard all do it in hope of fair advantage.

Shakespeare reminds us that risk is concerned not only with the possibility of loss or harm, but also with the hope of some benefit or gain.[1]

Contrast Shakespeare's concept of risk with the more popular notion of risk which involves primarily the negative aspect. Typical comments about the daredevil stuntman might include, "He's a fool; he's going to get himself killed"; rarely is it ever said, "What a daredevil! He's going to achieve fame and glory" and yet both outcomes, the negative or the posi-

Susan M. McFadden is an Occupational Therapy Consultant in Memphis, Tennessee. Bonnie Hanschu is Chairperson of Occupational Therapy, Cambridge State Hospital, Cambridge, Minnesota. The paper is adapted from one the authors wrote in *Australian Occupational Therapy Journal* after practicing in that country.

This article appears jointly in *Private Practice in Occupational Therapy* (The Haworth Press, Inc., 1985), and *Occupational Therapy in Health Care*, Volume 2, Number 2 (Summer 1985).

tive, are possible. The occupational therapist who takes a risk and reports unethical work behavior may be thought of in negative terms, such as "a tattler" or may be thought of as risking the chance of promotion; rarely does someone point out that this occupational therapist's risk behavior provides a valued service to the employer and the profession as a whole.

Similarly, risk takers are frequently thought of in negative terms. Risk takers are the gamblers, the boat rockers, and the fish who try to swim against the current. Sometimes they win, sometimes they stay afloat, and sometimes the current is too strong and sweeps them down the channel. However, we should realize that if they succeed, they will succeed big and the rewards will be great; if they lose they have the satisfaction of having tried, often gaining more than they lose by what they learn in the process.

Risk takers are also the explorers and discoverers of this world. They are among the creators and innovators who help find a new path, develop a better way, who help us get to a different and often advanced place in our thinking, doing, and understanding.

There are many examples of risk takers as creative innovators in occupational therapy—Reilly, Ayres, Weimer, and West to name a few. Surely, no one would argue with the notion that these people went out on a limb and that our profession benefited by their risk taking behaviors.

Risk arises in some form or other in virtually all areas of endeavor. Risk is a constant factor in our personal lives as well as in our professional lives. It is important neither to ignore risk nor to be frightened by it. Occupational therapists practice in the health care arena where many risks come from multifaceted and conflicting external sources. Today there is more pressure than ever before for us to contain our costs, validate our outcomes, and make our services accessible to those who need it most. Baum recognized the positive aspects of our changing health care arena and pointed out that *"The risks we take will lead to an even stronger identity for the occupational therapy profession."*[2, p 455]

With the realization that risk involves both negative and positive potential, we should consider adopting the concept of "risk management". This concept acknowledges that risk is a fact of life and therefore is not something which can be avoided, but rather managed in a creative way. Risk management includes incorporating that attitude into the decision making process. This can lead occupational therapists individually or the profession as a whole into carefully thought out risk situations in the hope of positive outcome, as opposed to always avoiding these risk situations because of their negative potential. In a 1981 article, the authors described risk taking as a process of going out on a limb. In articulating a risk taking attitude they described the need for frequent innovation and the weighing of reasonable risks against available alternatives in the hope of making timely and cost-effective services accessible.[3]

There are different areas in which we can address the need for progressive risk taking attitudes. Perhaps one of the most important ones is the educational arena. There is little evidence that as educators we are expressing the need for a risk taking attitude and incorporating the concept of that attitude into either student selection or curriculum development. Johnson, Arbes, and Thompson[4] in a survey of 32 educational programs, remarked that only one program volunteered the fact that they preferred risk taking attitudes in their prospective students. And why, you might ask, should we seek out risk takers for our educational programs? Theodore Roosevelt provides insight into that question by saying

> Far better it is to dare mighty things, to win glorious triumphs, even though checked by failure, than to take rank with those poor spirits who neither enjoy much nor suffer much, because they live in the gray twilight that knows neither victory or defeat.[5, p 15]

Occupational therapists have, over the years, developed strategies to deal with or reduce risks, but these strategies frequently involve avoidance. The teaching of positive risk taking strategies or risk management is not readily apparent in our educational programs nor in the continuing education programs for practicing therapists. Yet, several authors[3,6,7,8] have offered positive suggestions for learning how to deal with risks. Some of these suggestions include evaluating priorities, keeping risks in perspective, perfecting communication skills—both written and verbal, gathering as much information as possible, analyzing information, and systematically identifying alternatives. Perhaps competencies for occupational therapy education which are concerned with risk taking should include: (a) the ability to identify both negative as well as positive aspects of risk; and (b) the ability to apply the concept of risk management.

Three principle points are made: firstly, it is important to reach the understanding that risk involves the prospect of either negative or positive outcome; secondly, with that understanding in mind, one should adopt the concept of risk management which will lead one to enter into risk situations in the hope of positive outcome as opposed to always avoiding them because of their negative potential; thirdly, methods for dealing with risks have been identified and need to be taught.

> There is a tide in the affairs of men
> Which taken at the flood leads on to fortune;
> Omitted, all the voyage of their life
> Is bound in shallows and in miseries.
>
> William Shakespeare

REFERENCES

1. Moore PG: *The Business of Risk,* New York: Cambridge University Press, 1983

2. Baum CM: A Look at Our Strengths in the 80's: *Am J Occup Ther* 37:451–455, 1983

3. Hanschu B, McFadden SM: Out on a Limb: A Novel Approach for Traditional Occupational Therapy Practice. *Aust Occup Ther J* 28:39–46, 1981

4. Johnson RW, Arbes BH, Thompson CG: Selection of Occupational Therapy Students. *Am J Occup Ther* 28:597–601, 1974

5. Mueller RK: *Risk, Survival, and Power,* New York: American Management Association, 1970

6. Oliver ML: Taking Risks Will Get Your Career Moving. *Pers J* 62:318–320, 1983

7. Byrd RE: *A Guide to Personal Risk Taking,* New York: American Management Association, 1974

8. Fischhoff B et al: *Acceptable Risk,* New York: Cambridge University Press, 1981

Tidal Surge and Private Practice: The Historic Eighties

Betty Wild Frazian, OTR/L

ABSTRACT. There are historic changes occurring in American society and not least among them is a veritable transformation of the delivery of health care. Many circumstances, historical and economic, including a growing enlightenment among the public, are demanding innovation on a greater scale than ever before, and the private practitioner is responding with historic pervasive innovation.

When General Cornwallis surrendered to General Washington at Yorktown, his troops stacked arms before the ranks of the Colonials and his band struck up the march "When the World Turned Upside Down."

There is no band announcing to us the sweep of profound change in contemporary American society since the Sixties. We simply do not do most things as we used to and society pushes forward. Now society is pushing the structure of the delivery of health care with a tidal surge of change. Not the tug of the moon, but the carrot and stick of government, the wallet of the consumer, the awareness of the consumer, the advance of technology, are in effect, destabilizing and deinstitutionalizing the ways we deliver service to the patient.

Betty Wild Frazian is President of Health Professional Associates, P.O. Box 3526, Ormond Beach, FL 32074. HPA is a sole proprietorship group practice emphasizing specialized assessment, treatment and research in occupational therapy. Health Professional Seminars, a division of HPA, provides continuing education and training for therapists nationally and eventually internationally.

Mrs. Frazian was formerly creator of a pioneering group practice in Boston called Associated Occupational Therapists from 1968 to 1977. She is currently writing a book, *Private Practice for Health Professionals,* based on her experience and research in independent practice.

This article appears jointly in *Private Practice in Occupational Therapy* (The Haworth Press, Inc., 1985), and *Occupational Therapy in Health Care,* Volume 2, Number 2 (Summer 1985).

It is more than mere change; it is fast change and that makes all the difference.

SOCIETY DICTATES

Fast change has a logic and irony of its own. Merely a symptom and not a first cause of this fast change is the government's new cost-control strictures in Medicare which, in the short term, are reducing occupancy rates in hospitals and are expanding service to the outpatient. Private practice among physicians is declining; among other health care professionals it is increasing. The quality of health care can improve, often dramatically, under the ostensible duress of the ethic of efficiency. Society is tapping out a drumbeat of rapid change, and it is hoped that the good of the traditional remains whilst the good of new enterprise develops, both redounding to the benefit of the modern patient.

The fundamental question is, of course, what does society want? No institutional framework can long endure in a free society without adherence to the dictates of that society. In matters of health care delivery, society raised its voice through its elected representatives in 1965 with the promulgation of Medicare and Medicaid. Precedent was set against a hue and cry of socialized medicine.

THEN AND NOW

Such reaction was understandable, for it was a long way philosophically from the early days of medicine as a cottage industry when the physician took payment in cash or cordwood. It was even a long way from the Thirties in America when health insurance first began to spread its influence. There was time and space for philosophical debate then; there is little time and less space for that now as society seeks full entitlement to all the advantages of health care.

It is the age of the third-party payor and the smart machine and the smart patient and the exploding cost (hospital expenses are up 456% since 1970).[1] The chief actuary of the Social Security system in 1965 at the inception of Medicare, the man who should have known, Robert Myers, "guessed" that hospital cost increases would actually slow down.[2] Now, out of frustration as much as knowledge, the government is guessing that cost controls will alter the pattern of rising costs.[3] Aetna Life & Casualty Company calls these control efforts the most dramatic change in their business in the last 25 years.[4]

We shall see. Symptom is often confused with cause. The occupational therapist, as citizen, as health care provider, as staff or independent or combination, must perceive bright-eyed the future of his or her professional practice from the disquiet of the present state of matters.

THE NEW INDEPENDENT

The president of Harvard University, Derek Bok, does not couch his profound concern in subtle argument or philosophical disputation. "The blunt fact," he says in his 1984 annual report, "is that most students today are getting an education that is far too narrow to prepare them for the challenges that await them in their working lives."[5] They are not keeping pace, he says, with the "changes in the system for delivering and financing health care."[6] He cites public criticism and other pressures and notes the "stirrings of change" across the country as he appeals for learning that is "problem-based."[7]

In an equally urgent declaration, the Association of American Medical Colleges in its first major report on medical education since 1932 demands a new type of independent professional. In calm but acerbic language, the writers propose altering "the entire process of selecting undergraduates for medical school and of training them to deal with the needs of patients."[8] Their historic report indicts "stifling rote learning" that creates "passive recipients of information."[9] Instead, it calls for a "self-directed" student who seeks "independent study" and wants more responsibility for his "own learning" in order to become a "lifelong learner" of independence.[10] The report is entitled "Physicians for the Twenty-First Century."

A less gracious expression of this sense of urgency informing all levels of health care in this country comes from a medical director, "I think the traditional medical practice where the office is open from one to three on Mondays and Thursdays is over . . . People won't stand for that."[11]

THE AGE OF INNOVATION

Insurance companies are demanding that things not remain the same. "We are witnessing an unprecedented expansion of competition and innovation in an industry that in the past seemed tradition-bound and impervious to the forces of supply and demand," says CIGNA.[12]

Most people fear change. Even the slightest switch in daily routine can produce unease, says philosopher Eric Hoffer.[13] How many of us seek risk? Who can deny the comfort of a regular paycheck and "benefits"?

Yet anyone who has lived in America since the Sixties knows that change is more common than permanence in his life. And, with or without acknowledging it, one now lives largely by innovation and self-direction. It is manifest that the profession of occupational therapy as a component of the health care industry and of society must embrace the innovator. And the private practitioner, with risk and without much help from precedent, is already performing on the "problem-based" sharp edge of change and social mandate.

It is not easy. Do not count, it is said, on even the changes remaining the same. Economist Alan Greenspan makes a cogent case for caution.[14] Medicare's cost controls are simply not, though crafted, compatible with the dynamics of a large private enterprise system, he says, and bottlenecks, political problems and inflation will develop. Irresistible pressures, he maintains, will create exemptions and eventually the exemptions will become the system. It is "only a matter of time before the control system unravels."[15] He concludes "innovation . . . is now our best hope . . . "[16]

Another leading thinker on health care delivery Peter Drucker argues that rapid change will become more rapid as the number of old and very old people and the explosive advances in medicine and medical technology accelerate.[17] Drucker, like Greenspan, sees hope, not in controls, but in a "market-based" health care system.[18] This country, he says, has enjoyed astounding benefits of a massive entrepreneurial economy in the past 15 years while Europe has not and Europeans still look to the big established company or to government for their jobs and career opportunities.[19] European society, he says, discourages people, especially the educated young whereas American society is open to the new venture despite its risks and uncertainties.[20]

NEW ERA IN OCCUPATIONAL THERAPY

It is not surprising that the profession of occupational therapy itself is undergoing a rapid rate of change—and recognition. Its extraordinary versatility and consistency of standards have brought unsolicited attention to the eyes of decision-makers seeking quality of care and reduction of costs. Occupational therapy is fast becoming known as a friend to a growing society of smart patients and health care personnel who want delivery on their own terms.

It is certainly no accident or statistical aberration that the Bureau of Labor Statistics projects the growth of occupational therapy employment to fall within the top 20 occupations in the country between 1982 and 1995; thirteenth, to be exact, surpassing sixteenth place physical therapy.[21]

The articles which follow in this issue of *Occupational Therapy in Health Care* constitute an exciting in-depth sampling of innovation. And, as it should, practice is distancing theory, and "models" of practice are being created before they are defined. The empirical should always instruct the theoretical, and society's needs are occasioning combination and recombination in practice. Medicare and Medicaid did it. Public Law 94-142 in 1975 did it for public schools. Medicare's cost controls are doing it again. Pending legislation in Congress for inclusion of occupational therapy services under Part B of Medicare would further change combinations in health care delivery. There will be no foreseeable end to the list of variables in "setting" as innovative therapists increase in number to meet society's appetite. Unions, companies, health maintenance organizations, home health agencies, free-standing clinics, private payors, lawyers, state and insurance regulators, sports teams, physical health enthusiasts, want delivery of occupational therapy talent to the patient, the client, the courtroom, the coal mine.

BE PREPARED

Fast change is sending its summons to the private practitioner. The list will grow off the page. The moving finger will not stop and all compilations of statistics in an environment of fast change and fluid setting are suspect. Even the definition of private practice is disputed. There is the purely staff therapist and the purely independent therapist. And in between, there are uncounted occupational therapists who are designing lifestyles and professional practices to suit need, theirs and society's, in varying degrees of risk.

The independent-thinking therapist in the institutional setting and in private setting are fashioning a new model, if you will, of activism. There is a proliferation of specialty seminars and a cascade of guiding literature by therapists for therapists. It is the age of the specialist and of the vital mechanism of networking. Witness the hand therapists, for example, as they skillfully organize to help each other.

There is the ungrudging acceptance of the modern concomitants of riskful initiative practice, such as marketing, public relations, contractual agreements, office leases, personal insurance, billing complexity, competition, carrying inventory of supplies, equipment, and special individual pressure to maintain the highest standards.

CONCLUSION

Form follows function if unfettered. Society dispatched "reconstruction aides" in World War I to help the wounded in rehabilitation. Thenceforth, this nascent discipline began its evolution in theory and practice as the profession of occupational therapy in subsequent decades.

Change in the Eighties will be measured in months.

REFERENCES

1. Barbour J: Medical Industry Copes with Cost. *Daytona Beach Sunday News-Journal,* May 20, 1984, p. 1E

2. Fialka J: Candidates Avoid Medicare Cure. *Wall Street Journal,* September 12, 1984, p. 64

3. Ibid

4. Labor Letter. *Wall Street Journal,* September 18, 1984, p. 1

5. Fiske E: Harvard President Urges Changes in Training of American Doctors. *New York Times,* April 21, 1984, p. 1

6. Ibid

7. Ibid., p. 10.

8. Maeroff G: Medical Training Assailed by Panel. *New York Times,* September 20, 1984, p. 21

9. Ibid

10. Ibid

11. Smart T: Times Have Changed. *Miami Herald,* July 16, 1984, p. 11

12. Ibid

13. Hoffer E: The Ordeal of Change. New York: Harper & Row, 1963, p. 3

14. Greenspan A: Payment Set-up Can't Ensure Medicare's Fit. *Wall Street Journal,* September 4, 1984, p. 35

15. Ibid

16. Ibid

17. Drucker P: We Must Rethink Health Care Fundamentals. *Wall Street Journal,* July 5, 1984, p. 22

18. Ibid

19. Drucker P: Europe's High-Tech Delusion. *Wall Street Journal,* September 14, 1984, p. 24

20. Ibid

21. Dataline: OT Among Twenty Fastest Growing Occupations. *Occupational Therapy Newspaper,* March 1984, p. 6

Community Occupational Therapy Associates: A Model of Private Practice for Community Occupational Therapy

Karen Goldenberg, BSc(OT), OT(C)
Barbara Quinn, BSc(OT), OT(C)

ABSTRACT. This article describes the creation and evolution of an occupational therapy practice agency in Canada. It explains how the agency has grown to meet the needs of both patients and therapists, and gives case examples as illustrations of successful intervention.

Although Community Occupational Therapy Associates (Comm. O.T.) was born and has flourished in a Canadian climate, many of the principles implicit in its structure and process could be used anywhere. Indeed, Comm. O.T. may be described both as a model for community health care and as a response to our changing world. Comm. O.T. has operated since 1973 in Metropolitan Toronto, a city of 2-1/2 million people situated in the province of Ontario which is in the centre of Canada. Comm. O.T. demonstrates not only the principle of decentralized, non-institutional health care, but also the changing, expanding role that awaits occupational therapists willing to take up the challenge.

Karen Goldenberg is Executive Director, Barbara Quinn Assistant Director, and Fern Lebo, Staff Therapist, all of Community Occupational Therapy Associates, Toronto, Ontario, Canada.

The authors would like to acknowledge the editorial assistance of Fern Lebo, OT (C), Comm. OT.

This article appears jointly in *Private Practice in Occupational Therapy* (The Haworth Press, Inc., 1985), and *Occupational Therapy in Health Care*, Volume 2, Number 2 (Summer 1985).

15

COMM. O.T. FROM THE BEGINNING

Comm. O.T. growth from its birth until the end of 1983 shows dramatically how the program has caught fire. Such successful development has necessitated changes in Comm. O.T.'s organization and philosophy. However, throughout this rapid expansion, the group has tried to stay flexible, versatile and responsive.

The idea for Comm. O.T. began with five independent occupational therapists who were frustrated by their restrictive hospital settings. They were not able to follow-up their discharge patients adequately when they were forced to cope with the realities of daily living in their homes and their communities. These five therapists perceived a role evolving for community health workers who would assist individuals to develop the life skills needed to survive in a large complex bustling city like Toronto. It seemed crucial that someone should work with individuals in their own environments to discover their physical and psycho-social needs and to develop ways of satisfying them. Occupational therapists with their training and expertise in using activity to improve function to develop confidence, and to promote integrated activity, were ideal for filling this role.

The Ministry of Health of Ontario, which runs a provincially sponsored health insurance plan covering 99% of the population of the province, had been contemplating a home care program since the early 60's. Spiralling costs of hospital care had forced the government to consider alternate methods of treating persons with physical and psycho-social dysfunction. But consumers of health care were conditioned to go to hospital whether they needed treatment in this expensive setting or not. Questions being considered by government and treatment personnel alike were whether or not there were more humane and ultimately more successful methods of treating people in their own milieu. It was generally believed that better methods must exist.

The five occupational therapists who founded Comm. O.T. realized that they could play a vital role in the execution of this philosophy and be on the cutting edge of the expansion of their profession, taking it into new and exciting vistas.

Since occupational therapy outside institutions is not an

insured service in Ontario, a funding source was needed. The solution seemed to be to achieve a relationship with the Home Care Program of Metropolitan Toronto, a Ministry of Health agency, which was already coordinating services such as nursing, physiotherapy, speech therapy and homemaking. The five therapists formed a formal business partnership and presented a proposal which was accepted by the Home Care Program of Metropolitan Toronto (Home Care). Operation began on a small scale in June 1973. A purchase-of-service model was employed with a fee established based on a fixed rate-per-treatment. As the program evolved, an hourly rate was set, and Home Care was billed for the hours involved in a total treatment. Individual therapists who provided services were paid an hourly rate, which covered actual patient care, as well as time related to travel, reporting, recording and data gathering.

At the beginning, none of the five partners could be financially dependent on the program, and each continued with her full-time job or family responsibilities. An initial investment by each was made to cover the cost of malpractice insurance and administrative expenses. Many hours were spent developing and interpreting the role that occupational therapy could play in the community.

Soon, an explosion in the number of referrals necessitated locating and engaging more therapists to work in specific geographical areas of the city. The therapists were then, and still are, free-lance private practitioners, who commit themselves to work at Comm. O.T. at least 25 hours per week. At the end of 1977, there were 30 therapists working the equivalent of approximately 20 full-time positions.

By 1975, the partnership structure of Comm. O.T. was no longer suitable and incorporation into a non-profit corporation was implemented. A board of directors was formed, bringing in individuals with expertise in program planning, business practices, law, insurance, fiscal planning, and community health. The board now meets three times a year to review the total program and to determine policies. A financial committee manages the fiscal operation of organization and a program committee monitors ongoing programs and considers future expansion. Therapists employed now number close to 70, a full-time equivalency of more than 50.

The following examples demonstrate both the diversity of patients seen and the multiplicity of skills employed by the occupational therapist in effecting community adjustment of the patients.

CASE EXAMPLES

Case One

1. Elizabeth is a 32-year-old art student with a history of chronic schizophrenia. Her successful community re-integration shows how the revolving door syndrome associated with her condition can be arrested. Elizabeth was referred to Comm. O.T. by a general practitioner via Home Care. Previous treatment programs included multiple hospitalizations, E.C.T., drug and megavitamin therapy. She was an unkempt, malnourished, disoriented woman who was sleeping 16 to 18 hours per day, hallucinating and unable to cope with her life in the community.

Occupational therapy goals were to improve Elizabeth's skills in hygiene, dressing, and diet; to establish routines for taking her medication; to teach her how to prepare meals; and to budget her time, and her finances. Further goals were to re-establish her school routines and to reduce her social isolation. Other services involved were Homemaking early in the treatment program and later Public Health Nursing for follow-up. Over a 3-1/2 month period 26 visits were made by the occupational therapist with gradual withdrawal of visits during the last 6 weeks.

By the time of discharge, Elizabeth was attending art classes and had established a regular routine of diet and medication. Also she has moved to more suitable housing, and was attending both Yoga classes and an exercise group at the Y.W.C.A. A follow-up after 2-1/2 years revealed that Elizabeth was managing in the community with intermittent contact from her family practitioner and Public Health Nurse. There had been no rehospitalizations.

Case Two

2. Mrs. S. is a 68-year-old widow living in a nursing home, severely disabled from a stroke. She was referred to Comm.

O.T. by a physiotherapist and a staff physician via Home Care. Five years earlier a cerebral vascular accident had left her with a right hemiplegia and expressive aphasia. Previous treatment had included a short stay in a general hospital and five months in a convalescent hospital. At that time, she appeared to be unable to benefit from rehabilitation due to poor motivation and a denial of her illness. She was a depressed, withdrawn woman, wheelchair-bound and dependent in all activities of daily living.

The occupational therapy goals were: improvement in her self-care skills in dressing, eating and hygiene; ambulation and independent transfers; and participation in social activities in the Home. Other services were provided by a speech therapist and the nursing home staff. Forty visits by the occupational therapist over a five month period were made as part of a comprehensive treatment program.

On discharge, Mrs. S. was walking independently with one cane; eating, dressing, transferring independently, and bathing with supervision. She was taking part in group activities in the Home, going on outings with her friends, and generally re-establishing contact with the outside community.

Case Three

3. Tom is a 44-year-old man with paraplegia confined for 6 years to a chronic care hospital. His return into the community after this prolonged stay is an exciting example of rehabilitation. Tom was referred by a hospital neurologist via Home Care. Following a car accident while intoxicated, Tom was left with high level paraplegia and his rehabilitation was complicated by much denial of his condition, hostility and self-abuse. Chronic pressure sores, fused hips, and uncooperative behaviour caused many difficulties in his course of treatment.

Tom was an unhappy man apparently destined to live in an institution although he wanted very much to live outside on his own. A team conference in hospital which included the patient, a Home Care co-ordinator and the Comm. O.T. therapist facilitated a realistic assessment and the development of a treatment plan which would enable Tom to try to return to the community.

The occupational therapy program included teaching homemaking and household management skills; establishing routines and procedures of personal care; modification of his home setting with many aids and adaptations in the bathroom and kitchen; linking Tom with community services for home help. Tom received 18 occupational therapy visits over a 2-1/2 month period. A visiting nurse provided daily treatment for the chronic bed sores and the occupational therapist was able to provide ongoing follow-up after the initial 10 weeks, through the Comm. O.T. Mental Health Aftercare Program.

A follow-up visit one year later, found Tom continuing to live alone in his apartment. He can also be seen bumping up a curb with a case of beer on his wheelchair or at the local racetrack which has wheelchair access.

These cases admittedly are somewhat typical; but illustrate the variety and complexity of caseload. The average length of stay on the program is 31 days, and the average number of visits per patient is 10.

COMMUNITY OCCUPATIONAL THERAPY AS A MODEL

The provision of occupational therapy in a community setting is exciting, realistic and satisfying. The broad concept of a private enterprise selling direct service and consultation to a variety of health and social agencies has many advantages and could be adapted to suit many contexts. The model is flexible enough to change, expand or contact, according to current demands. It also offers the freedom to anticipate and to develop expanding roles for occupational therapy in the growing field of community health. Sub-contracting with free-lance private practitioners brings much-needed personnel into the work force, at the same time enabling individuals with other interests or responsibilities to work within a flexible time frame. This maximizes benefits to patients as well since such therapists can provide visits in the daytime, the evenings or on weekends, according to need.

The program attracts independent, mature confident therapists who may set and vary their own work schedules, thereby encouraging and facilitating the development of creative, resourceful professionals.

Comm. O.T. provides a central, friendly office which handles referrals and finances, provides supervision, consultation and in-service training, as well as equipment and supplies, not to mention the annual Christmas party. One of the many challenges experienced by community occupational therapists, as well as other community workers, is the isolation of working alone in a non-structured environment. Comm. O.T. has encouraged the formation of a therapists' council which gives therapists an opportunity to meet at least once a month for mutual support and the exchange of information and ideas.

Comm. O.T. has been accepted enthusiastically by consumers, purchasing agencies, and other individuals and services involved in community health care. In spite of general fiscal restraints in health care services, Comm. O.T. has continued to grow (Figures 1 and 2). Recently, direct funding

ADMISSIONS AND TREATMENTS

1973 - 1982

A Ten Year Comparision

Year	No. of Pts. Admitted	No. of Treatments
1973	173	527
1974	487	2,252
1975	854	4,340
1976	1,453	9,517
1977	2,386	16,392
1978	2,996	21,425
1979	3,191	25,215
1980	3,621	28,875
1981	4,535	37,542
1982	4,315	35,992

Figure 1

COMMUNITY OCCUPATIONAL THERAPY ASSOCIATES

THERAPIST DEPLOYMENT

Year	Number of Therapists	Full Time Equivalent
1973	5	.8
1974	9	2.5
1975	12	4
1976	16	8
1977	30	20
1978	34	24
1979	39	28
1980	53	30
1981	63	40
1982	68	42

Figure 2

was received to develop a long-term follow-up program for psychiatric patients, now called the Mental Health Aftercare Program. Comm. O.T. has also received funding to support a social network therapy program for chronic psychiatric patients and a new volunteer program which a therapist administers.

RESULTS

A sustained effort to measure the effectiveness of Comm. O.T. services has led to the development of a sophisticated research proposal to evaluate the results achieved thus far with mental health patients. A 3-year Demonstration Model grant has just been received from the Ontario Ministry of Health to implement this research plan.

The experience of Community Occupational Therapy Associates in Toronto has shown that occupational therapists can take their place at the leading edge of progress in community health. Members of the profession have the skills, the talents and the inclination to adapt and to contribute to the changing demands of providing health care. The challenge is there. The staff at Comm. O.T. hope to encourage others to grasp it.

A New Arena for Private Practice in Occupational Therapy: Worker's Compensation and Personal Injury

Doris J. Shriver, OTR

ABSTRACT. The "occupational therapist in private practice" during the last decade seems to be an expected topic for conventions, task forces and cocktail clutches among therapists. Manuals have been published, seminars given and a list of consultants has been made available for those asking the big question "Should I set up my own practice?" Still, the letters and phone calls persist. "How do I start?" Occupational therapist's nonetheless now are numerous in the private sector and represent many different models of practice. The intent of this article is to introduce the role and function of the private practice occupational therapist in evaluation, treatment, consultation and testimony for worker's compensation or personal injury cases. The definition of private practice for this paper is a sole proprietorship, staffed by independent contracting therapists providing direct services in the private practice office. Certain aspects of business administration will also be included.

To have a "private practice" is an idea that crosses the minds of most occupational therapists at one time or another since the private practice setting provides a unique opportunity for individual therapists to profit from their skills *and* better control their professional destiny. As the trend for health care is expanding services away from the institutional

Doris J. Shriver is Owner and Director of a free-standing Private Practice in Denver, Colorado. She was instrumental in developing the AOTA guidelines for Private Practice and continues to contribute to the development of standards in this area of professional activity.

This article appears jointly in *Private Practice in Occupational Therapy* (The Haworth Press, Inc., 1985), and *Occupational Therapy in Health Care*, Volume 2, Number 2 (Summer 1985).

25

setting so is the trend of the occupational therapist toward the private practice model. Before one should anticipate the promise of new arenas of practice, components of the business itself must first be considered.

A PRIVATE PRACTICE AS A BUSINESS

Although the occupational therapist is well trained to provide services unique to the profession the complexity of starting and running a business requires skills for which the occupational therapist is ill-prepared. The "business" serves as a foundation from which the therapist provides services and, therefore, must be managed and operated with expertise. The first order of business for an occupational therapist who is anticipating the adventure of private practice, or for the occupational therapist already in private practice who can not seem to get "over the hump", is to review the AOTA manual on Private Practice.[1] For those who may feel they do not need it, or who plan to order the manual later, an outline of the major topics in the manual is listed to show the great scope of concerns that must be addressed in establishing and operating a successful private practice.

I. BUSINESS MANAGEMENT

    A. Promoting practice
        —Location
        —Referral
        —Advertising and Public Relations
        —Health Care Trends

    B. Banking and Financing
        —Initial Capital
        —Loan Structuring and Resources
        —Bank Accounts
        —Grants

    C. Office Lay-out and Design
        —Space
        —Supplies and Equipment
        —Design

D. Office Systems and Procedures
 —Record Keeping
 —Filing
 —Billing
 —Policy and Procedures
 —Forms
 —Safety-Emergency Procedures
 —Office Communication
 —Office Controls

E. Solo vs. Group

F. Contracts and Agreements

G. Personnel Management
 —Hiring/Firing
 —Training
 —Supervision
 —Employee Review
 —Management Systems

H. Insurance

I. Expense and Overhead Control
 —Disbursement System/Control
 —Budget
 —Fee Schedule
 —Taxes

II. Legal Information

III. Third Party Reimbursement

IV. Quality Assurance

V. AOTA Standards, Guidelines, Policies, Etc.

VI. Professional Development

Your business *must* address every one of these organizational and operating aspects in detail applying the highest standards available, if you are to plan and operate successfully. One should gather information by attending seminars, getting literature from the U.S. Small Business Administration and business consultation agencies, taking relevant classes, and hiring consultation from accountants, attorneys, financial experts, and peers. Expect to pay for these professional services and in order to make such sessions productive have specific questions ready. Your approach in using resources must be professional and well planned. If you find that no one wants to help you, begin again, you probably are not yet adequately prepared to use the help available.

"Prepared" means that you have explored your options and are familiar with the implications of a variety of possibilities of structure and operation. For example, you might have a list of the legal points, that are available from any public library, that should be contained in a contract for consultation (i.e., services, fees, payments, liability, taxes, termination) but, you need advice about how to protect yourself from an employee that might start sub-contracting with your referral sources. In other words, take the time to identify your needs and problems and frame your questions before you seek consultation. If you begin a consulting session with "do I need a contract to provide services or to hire consultants?", what you are really saying, is that you do not really know what you are attempting, and want someone else to make your important decisions. A potential advisor is more apt to help someone who appears more ready to be independent and successful.

Along with organization and operational planning the second ingredient of a business is the *product*. The best laid plans for operating and managing a business are useless unless the product and/or services are also *specific* and of the highest quality. Know your craft well, have ready at hand the literature and research that supports your theories, hire capable staff that strengthen the quality of services offered and give evidence by documented certification of your skills whenever possible. Your confidence in yourself and your ability as an occupational therapist has to be strong because you will not have time to relearn therapy skills as you struggle with day to day operational demands.

Once you have combined a good plan for the business management with a strong, saleable product, you are ready to go. It sounds simple enough. But, now you have to accept that you may not make a profit for from one to three years, with work weeks of an average of 80 hours even while health care trends and new laws possibly dissipate your market. However, if your professional skills and relentless desire to succeed do not wane, once well launched you will always have a foundation from which to develop another market and mold a product to meet new needs.

WORKER'S COMPENSATION
AND PERSONAL INJURY TODAY

A rapidly emerging arena for the practice of occupational therapy is in vocational rehabilitation for persons involved in worker's compensation or personal injury situations. Although occupational therapists in hospital settings are often initially involved with this client the profession in general has been sadly remiss for not continuing its involvement after acute care stages by emphasizing and reinforcing its heritage in return to work concerns. The constraints of the medical model and the professions' trend toward specialization seems to have stunted growth and expansion into this now viable market. Occupational therapists have not been providing the physician, the insurance industry, the attorney, nor the injured worker with the information that they need to understand and facilitate the "return to work process". Therefore, usually the physician and the private vocational counselor are left to determine how the client can best function in a particular job. Yet neither has the skills in functional evaluation and treatment that the occupational therapist does. According to a professor of vocational rehabilitation at a local university, if occupational therapists had not become specialized and confined themselves to the hospitals, there would not be rehabilitation counselors.

The industry that centers on worker's compensation and personal injury is crying out for qualified experts in the private sector who are qualified to assist in rehabilitation. Physicians, vocational counselors, work evaluators, attorneys, claims adjusters and judges trying injury cases need clear, meaningful and objective information regarding the current and projected functional status of the injured client. The physician is hard pressed to make decisions regarding a client's ability to return to his previous occupation. He often must make decisions based solely on information from standard "Guides" to rating physical impairment which do not take into consideration the client's actual disability. An amputation of the dominant index finger, for example, carries the same impairment rating for the construction worker as it does for the legal secretary. The actual impairment may be the same but the disability may be far more serious for the legal secretary who must have discreet function of fingers of both hands to do her work. Some physicians are now refusing to rate physical impairment for litigation in insurance cases because they feel they are being asked by the legal system to make judgments beyond their areas of expertise.[2]

Many laws for state worker's compensation and personal injury now make vocational rehabilitation services mandatory as part of the services for workers who are injured or as a component of the major medical policy for personal injuries. This change has given rise to the establishment of numerous private rehabilitation agencies and consultants, each claiming that they provide "the ultimate in rehabilitation". Although these "rehabilitationists" are providing valuable services in many cases, there is growing conflict among those in this emerging industry, and between them and the agencies/individuals that require their services. Free enterprise is not always conducive to functioning with the controls nor the standards and ethics that a consumer with a disability has come to expect. A client frequently feels that the "rehabilitationist" has compromised his, the client's, position in favor of the insurance company. Persons from the insurance industry say that the "rehabilitationist" has in many cases abused fees and could have done a better job. The physician thinks that the "rehabilitationist" does not understand and in fact violates the patient-doctor relationship and that eagerness to place the disabled client on a job sometimes takes precedence over the client's general welfare.[3] State consumer protection agencies are concerned that "rehabilitationists" may not be adequately qualified and regulated. Some of these kinds of professional conflicts have generated law suits and are currently being resolved in court.

THE OCCUPATIONAL THERAPIST PROVIDING VOCATIONAL REHABILITATION SERVICES

The neophyte rehabilitation counselor in the private sector is facing the same identity crisis that occupational therapists faced over a decade ago. That crisis in occupational therapy brought about the development of Standards of Practice, Principles and Ethics, Due Process Procedures for Censure, Licensure, Uniform Terminology, Relative-Unit Values for Fees, Uniform Evaluation Procedures and numerous position papers and statements confirming and defining the scope and arena of occupational therapy practice.

Because the occupational therapist is registered (certified), and often licensed, has graduated from an educational program which is accredited, and has taken course content that speaks clearly to an understanding of human function in daily activities, including work, the occupational therapist is seen as an expert in the field of vocational rehabilitation.

An occupational therapist, thanks to the standard settings efforts of the professional association, is now better prepared than ever to step into the arena of private rehabilitation using well documented procedures and tools. For the first time, therapists have an opportunity to help define the commonly accepted purpose of rehabilitation (return to daily work) and to make significant changes to improve services to this end in the private sector.

Some agencies specializing in rehabilitation use the services of many professionals: vocational counselors, work evaluators, physicians, psychologists, social workers, rehabilitation nurses, and ancillary therapists and programs, a not unusual team composition. Having been reared in the medical model setting, most occupational therapists, it seems, should have little difficulty adjusting to such collegiality in the private rehabilitation community. Unfortunately, however, the team approach has not been widely accepted outside of hospitals and competition among services in the private sector is so fierce that the newly arrived private occupational therapy practitioner can be viewed as another competitor rather than as a welcome and useful ingredient to everyone's success. For this reason, as a private practice occupational therapist, one may not be able initially to develop easily referral sources in the rehabilitation community. One may, however, make a first appearance as a consultant or as an expert witness at the request of an attorney representing either the plaintiff or the defendant in a workers compensation or personal injury suit who needs objective answers to questions such as:

1. Why does the claimant's injury affect his ability to return to work, perform daily tasks or participate in leisure activities?
2. Is vocational rehabilitation for the claimant appropriate? And, if so, what considerations and/or adaptations should be considered to make him job functional?
3. Is the claimant using the disability for secondary gains?
4. Does pain affect the claimant's physical functional skills and/or activities of daily living?
5. Does the claimant have residual functional skills that can be used to identify transferable abilities?

These are difficult questions whenever asked, but they must be answered and must reflect compliance with state laws that govern litigation of worker's compensation or personal injury cases. The occupational therapist is uniquely qualified to provide services that shed a new perspective on the issues of functional loss and rehabilitation potentials by giving service in the areas of evaluation, program planning, treatment, consultation and testimony.

EVALUATION

The functional areas of activities of daily living, sensorimotor skills, cognitive skills, psycho-social skills, and the need for therapeutic aids and/or adaptations as well as the ability to practice prevention skills (body mechanics, work simplifications, etc.), should be thoroughly examined. To do this the occupational therapy evaluation process should include the use of standardized, non-standardized, and clinical assessments as well as observation and interview techniques.[4] The evaluation process thus administered can be conducted so that:

1. Subjective and objective data can be compared to either identify a potential malingerer or bring legitimacy to a client's dysfunction.
2. When a job or home site evaluation is combined with the clinical evaluation one can define the client's specific abilities or inabilities to perform required tasks.

3. Predictions based on standardized norms can be made regarding future losses in terms of wages on the job or contributions to the home.

The results from this assessment when combined with a review of the client's personal history, which includes developmental, educational, vocational, socio-economic as well as medical information, enables the therapist to provide objective data and to render an objective opinion regarding the client's status. These data may be presented to an economist who can attach dollar values to losses and the appropriate compensation can therefore be determined.

TREATMENT PROGRAMS

From the results of the occupational therapy evaluation a treatment program may be recommended. For example, an effective treatment program to improve range of motion, increase strength, reduce pain, develop endurance or improve body mechanics for the purpose of returning to work or increasing daily activities could uncover for the client opportunities that would otherwise not be considered.

An occupational therapist can design a graded program, for example, to monitor a client's daily activities, provide work hardening and manage his pain. Programming also can include adaptations for the work setting or operations, body mechanics training, pacing, and/or the prescription of assistive devices. Effective treatment truly requires looking at the whole person in order to provide effective service. It calls upon the widest range of skills of the therapist from her knowledge of medication to psycho-socio-cultural understandings. Few other service arenas demand as total a range of an occupational therapist's skills. Few, if any, other disciplines offer such a scope of perspectives.

CONSULTATION

Consultation might be provided to any one or all of the other professionals involved with the client and may be the most difficult aspect of providing services. Providing unbiased, professional consultation, while holding the client's best interest as a primary objective, is imperative. Knowledge or lack of knowledge of applicable laws, professional ethics and diplomatic strategies can be the difference between success and failure because of the multi professional arena that represents conflicting points of views about how to solve the often very complex nature of a given situation.

For example, consultation is provided to the vocational counselor who is usually in charge of developing the vocational rehabilitation plan; he needs to know the client's physical tolerances and functional skills. Consultation is also provided to the insurance claims adjustor who needs to know if a claimant needs more medical services or is ready for rehabilitation. The attorney wants to know if his client is disabled or not, and if so, to what degree. The physician wants to know if his patient would benefit from therapy or if he can go back to work. The client and his family wants to know "what's wrong with me?" and what might be in store for the future. Finally, consultation in the form of testimony as an expert witness might be requested from any one of these sources.

TESTIMONY

Professional testimony in the court or hearing room, or in the form of deposition, is accepted only after an occupational therapist has been qualified and accepted by the judge. Acceptance is based on educational background, professional experience, numbers of years in practice, numbers of clients with the disorders in question treated by the therapist, and certifiable skills in administering the tests and measurements being used to make judgments. Therapists wishing to qualify as experts may need to supply information such as transcripts and content of applicable courses from accredited curriculums attended along with complete resumes. On occasion the therapist may be asked to demonstrate a component of her skills for the court.

In addition to demonstrating personal qualifications, one

must be able to provide an understandable definition of occupational therapy thus setting the tone and scope of one's testimony. A definition suitable for a court often includes an historical perspective of the profession from its inception, its educational standards, to the profession's current inclusions in health care legislation. Relating treatment philosophy with a description of what an occupational therapist does is a common procedure.

The process of relating the results of the evaluation to the judge and jury should be reviewed with the presenting attorney before giving testimony. The therapist often must first educate the attorney who may or may not be representing the client. Many attorneys even ask that the therapist submit to them a list of likely questions about the client and his abilities so that during testimony the purpose and end result of the evaluation and its various components follows a logical and believable order. Cross-examination, which usually is an attempt to discredit the qualifications of the witness and invalidate the tests and/or the results presented, requires clear well thought out answers to questions that should be anticipated. One must express the results and/or final opinion in an unbiased and confident manner. Above all, the best interests of the client should never be compromised by an occupational therapist's testimony.

SUMMARY

Private practice is a growing dimension of occupational therapy services. A private practice requires not only a solid product but an efficient and effective business structure from which to operate. A particularly fast growing need for occupational therapy is in the arena of worker's compensation or personal injury. The occupational therapist by virtue of training has particular potential to provide a needed service in this private sector. Although the skills to manage such a business and provide these specific services is demanding, the potential is there and the market is ready. Some aspects of the function of the occupational therapist in this area of private practice have been reviewed and suggestions given.

REFERENCES

1. American Occupational Therapy Association, Practice Division: *Private Practice.* AOTA: (1383 Piccard Drive, Suite 300) Rockville, Maryland 20850 1982

2. Anderson, EM: The vocational evaluator—A new expert witness. *Trial Talk* Colorado Trial Lawyers Association, 31: 6, June 1982

3. Petrangelo GT, Abeln KE, Rudrub EH: Qualified rehabilitation consultants, how are they doing? *Vocational Evaluation and Work Adjustment Bulletin,* Spring 1984

4. Shriver, Mitcham, Schwartzberg, Ranucci: *Uniform Occupational Therapy Evaluation Checklist.* American Occupational Association—Commission on Practice, 1981

One Person's Experience in Private Practice: Start to Finish

Barbara M. Knickerbocker, OTR, FAOTA

ABSTRACT. This article will focus in a very personal way on a practice, its organization and composition, and on the procedures initiated in closing this large, full-time occupational therapy program. The practice has dealt exclusively with the treatment of childhood learning disorders, as well as with adolescents and adults identified under the current nomenclature of Attention Deficit Disorders.

Because the author was one of the first, if not *the* first, to establish a private practice in the treatment of learning disabilities, it is felt that all therapists can benefit from her unique personal experiences. The author cites what, in retrospect, might have been done differently, and offers concrete suggestions for therapists in establishing, maintaining and terminating a private practice in occupational therapy.

The driving force behind my decision to establish a private practice was the desire to do a detailed study of my clinical observations of the way children learned, and why some children had more difficulty learning. I knew I needed a milieu devoid of administrative distractions. My practice was one of the first—perhaps the only one of its kind for a number of years—functioning as a full-time, independent, self-supportive,

Barbara M. Knickerbocker founded The Princeton Center for Learning Disorders in Princeton, N.J., in 1966, one of the first private, parent-oriented research programs for the treatment of learning disabled children. Previously, she had served in the Army, developing a model program for training therapists in this field. She is the author of *A Holistic Approach to the Treatment of Learning Disorders* (1980). Ms. Knickerbocker has recently relocated to Vermont, where she plans to expand her work with adult patients.

This article appears jointly in *Private Practice in Occupational Therapy* (The Haworth Press, Inc., 1985), and *Occupational Therapy in Health Care,* Volume 2, Number 2 (Summer 1985).

research-oriented private practice for the treatment of learning disorders.

When I started in 1966, private practice for occupational therapists was uncommon; there were no precedents to follow nor role models, and there was skepticism in the therapeutic community about this new professional role. A few therapists around the country had begun to work independently, especially in Michigan, where some were working under the aegis of a child neurologist in Detroit. Following a tutorial model, they worked in their own homes with children after school, to supplement the family income. A smaller group was treating children with learning disorders as an adjunct to other employment.

Today, there are well-documented guidelines[2] to inform therapists about the need for legal services and to provide business advice before starting a private practice. There is no substitute for sound planning, research, consultation with others, and some attempt to assess the marketplace.

ESTABLISHING A PRIVATE PRACTICE[1]

Referrals

Therapists may find it advantageous not to immediately establish their own private practice, but rather provide the same services under the auspices of an established pediatric physician group. This builds a sound foundation for referrals for your private practice, when you decide to go out on your own, and suggests to other pediatricians that you have a "seal of approval."

There is another, perhaps hidden, benefit that comes from working with a pediatric group. It enables the therapist to develop good professional liaisons with one or more members of the local medical community who could be available on an informal basis—or as paid consultants—to discuss and advise on difficult situations within the realm of their training and orientation. This is especially important for young therapists who are apt to idealize being on their own, hoping to prove themselves through private practice.

The emotional focus on the Equal Rights Amendment and

the current glorification of entrepreneurism suggest to occupational therapists that private practice provides an answer for their own personal and professional goals. Any therapist planning to open a private practice must be totally realistic, and seriously consider the breadth of responsibility being undertaken. The problems inherent in legal, financial, safety, and security aspects of a private practice often surface only after the fact. Presumably, treating the patient, for which you are professionally trained, will give the least problems.

Another route toward building a future private practice could be to work in a school system, to establish a working relationship with people who can see the immediate value of your services. Unfortunately, teachers usually do not make recommendations to parents to seek private services for fear that the parents will hold the school system responsible for financial support. However, the ripple effect—by unofficial word-of-mouth communication in the community—can be helpful.

The best referrals come from satisfied parents. They can refer you to other parents who have a positive attitude and commitment to therapy, parents who are more likely to recognize the depth of their child's learning problems. Word-of-mouth from satisfied parents is your most important asset.

Advertising in the local papers brought only one referral after three months of weekly advertising. However, a feature article on two different occasions was a huge success. After one article appeared, there were thirty-five referrals, some coming even a year later.

The most effective approach that I discovered to generate a sound referral base was to offer courses about learning disorders in local adult education programs, the YWCA, or to parent groups affiliated with nursery schools or religious organizations. My first venture followed the ten-week protocol of the adult-education program; it was too long, by far. Since then, I have offered mini-courses of 3 or 4 two-hour sessions. Among these, the most successful was held in a public school where the program director was so eager for the community to be better informed about learning disabilities, he sent notices home with every child and urged teachers to attend. He priced the course to attract the public, at $3.00; seventy-five people attended. Remuneration for such courses is small, but the ultimate yield can be tremendous. Referrals from this broad exposure are still filtering in three years later.

I have conducted discussion groups in other schools for adults who have learning disorders, or are concerned that they, or someone they know, may have one. One year, I presented a series of morning programs to young mothers at the YWCA on early recognition and prevention of learning disorders. This was attended by twenty mothers, but yielded no referrals. Radio programs in two different years also proved ineffective.

When starting in a private practice, it could be helpful to set up your own "five-year plan." Consider different kinds of promotions, and what best fits your resources in terms of time, energy, and money. Courses take lots of time and energy, but no outlay of money. Mailing announcements that you are opening a practice is suitable, and takes relatively little time plus the cost of putting and mailing, but has marginal lasting impact. If you plan to give courses, determine where to focus your efforts to attain the best receptivity. For instance, Princeton is oriented more toward the educational approach, through special education tutoring; a few miles away, where my largest course was given, I found parents more receptive to a therapeutic approach. Repetition of a course in the same community in a second year does not yield as much as moving out to another satellite area. Do not be afraid of distance; if you have what people need, they will get there, even if it means driving their child an hour or more for therapy.

Since remuneration for any course is small, it is wise to consider it as building your long-range referral base; you are also providing service to the community. Since courses can drain your private time and energy, you must be selective. I offer at my own expense one-time lectures for religious organizations. However, for organizations—such as schools—that are gaining knowledge and information to improve their own performance, I charge my usual consultation fee.

Establishing Income Minimums

In any small operation, solving the cash-flow problem is crucial to success and survival. Before you start, you must have reasonable concept of how much your overhead will be, and the minimum number of clinical sessions per week necessary to break even. In my case, the break-even point was an average of seventeen hours per week; below that I would be subsidizing my own therapy program. For the purpose of calculating income, I use a forty-week year as a rule of thumb, but a fifty-two week year for determining operating expenses. The forty-week year—at five days a week—balances out earning time lost on vacations, holidays, snow days, and illness.

Cancellation Policy

In a private practice involving children, time lost due to illness of the child, the parent who drives the child, or other children in the family which prevents the parent from coming, can become a significant economic factor. As a therapist, you have to decide in advance various ways to handle this loss of income. It is usually not possible to fill the treatment appointment on short notice, but your overhead continues; your income can be devastated by a "flu" or chicken pox epidemic.

It took me a long time to come to grips with this problem. In an effort to keep it under control, I posted this sign in my office in clear view: "If an appointment is cancelled with less than twenty-four hours notice, there will be a charge." It didn't say the full charge, and I usually didn't enforce it, but it put the family on notice not to cancel unless absolutely necessary. A car breakdown, whether real or otherwise, is usually handled by trying to set up an alternate appointment during the same week, or by scheduling two appointments in the following week.

Gradually you get to know who abuses the policy, and then you may have to enforce it. It is a delicate matter, and I have found the few times that I tried to enforce it, one of two things happened: Either the family didn't cancel again, or, in one instance, the family stopped treatment. If there is some question in my mind about whether a cancellation is valid, I respond in this way: "I'm sorry you won't be able to make it. I would hate to have to bill you for this hour." Generally, the family will make new arrangements on the spot to attend that day or they will accept a make-up appointment. Because these problems occur, it is important at the end of the initial evaluation—if you are recommending therapy—that you clarify that you are holding this appointment time on a regular weekly basis, and what your cancellation policy is.

Seasonal Effects

Seasonal changes can also affect your operational income. I found, for instance, although September is a busy month for everyone, in private practice it can be very slow; people who were on summer vacation may not get around to resuming their treatment routine until October. I protected my economic status in two ways. When a child was leaving for the summer, I asked the parents if they wanted the same therapy time in the fall, giving them priority over patients just entering the program. The time would be tentatively reserved for the parents to confirm in late August, and therapy would resume after Labor Day.

The other change that I made was not to shut down for the month of August, as I was accustomed to doing. Any time there is a vacation or holiday break, there will be some disruption to the steady rhythm of the program. It is preferable to have an assistant to carry your program during absences. If you shut down the operation for a month, it is difficult to build up the same momentum; the loss of income in the following weeks can be substantial. As another countermeasure, I tried to increase my load in August to carry over into the fall program.

To assure a minimum loss of time, there is one policy that I should have set up but failed to do. When appointments are scheduled for evaluations a few weeks in advance, a follow-up call to reconfirm the appointment should be made the week before as a helpful reminder to the parents. This would also be helpful for patients who come for appointments infrequently. It assures the therapist that the time is either filled or, if the parents have decided to cancel, gives ample time to schedule another appointment. Nothing is quite so distressing as to rush to make an early morning appointment, and then wait and wonder.

Fee Payment Plans/Collections

Although I did not do so in the beginning, I found that I had to go to a pay-as-you-go plan, or my outstanding receipts built up and the cash-flow problem was unmanageable. Particularly when interest rates were high, I was, in effect, financing a patient's treatment if I waited to receive payment. I found that there were other merits to this alternate procedure. When the child has clearly had a productive session, the parents feel good and have a sense of relief about the child's problems; they pay more easily at the moment than when the fees accumulate over a month or two. Until I went on the pay-as-you-go-plan, I found parents would become embarassed when the bill was overdue; on occasion, this would cause the family to discontinue therapy.

Outstanding bills, which cannot be collected after personal reminders and ample discussion, are placed in the hands of a local Medical Service Bureau for collection. Most of the problems have been resolved by the pay-as-you-go plan that I have used during the past six years. I also accept VISA and Mastercard if necessary, but it is rarely needed; once you set the expectation for payment when services are rendered, the parents respond. Most importantly, good therapy must not be undermined by an emotional cloud of unpaid bills.

Billing/Fees

It is not unusual for occupational therapists to face some personal conflict about their worth in dollars and cents for the services that they provide. It is often difficult to raise fees. Here are a few guidelines that I found helpful. Fees should be increased at a clearly defined time, such as the beginning of a new school year, or a new calendar year, or at the beginning of the summer program. There may be children phasing out of the program, and lots of new referrals at those times. It is my usual policy not to raise the fee for those who will drop from the program within one or two months.

If the fee will be higher in the fall, I indicate to the parents before they leave for the summer what the increase will be. It is easiest to raise your fees by starting with those who are best able to pay them, or those whose financial burden is greatly eased by their insurance coverage. I have accepted some families for therapy at an agreed-upon fee which was lower than the going rate. I did not increase their fee over several years, because of their circumstances.

For third-party payment, I have two policies: (1) the parents pay me directly and then are reimbursed by their insurance company; and (2) I fill out my portion of the insurance form and always return it to the parents. It clearly becomes their responsibility to follow through; they also see exactly what I have written on their form. I always recommend that they have a physician co-sign the form, to avoid any delay or possible rejection by their insurance company.

I have learned over the years that insurance companies want a simple, brief, easily comprehensible statement; in contrast, an erudite professional treatise may be rejected. The problem has been made easier now by the American Psychiatric Association's classification of learning disorders of children and adults as Attention Deficit Disorders. These disorders carry a numerical medical identification which insurance companies recognize.[3]

Records and Reports

From habit developed in the Army, I started from the beginning to keep data for both *monthly* and *annual reports*. Although its format has changed over the years, each conveys a clear picture of growth, change, and details which years later provides useful information. I found it was also extremely helpful to have a narrative report to include: evaluations of patients by name and their referral source; business changes; visitors to the program; and all other professional activities, including lectures, courses or conferences I either attended or presented, and professional writing.

For a number of years, I have used the time-efficient Safeguard Business System for record keeping. With it one enters patient data by carbon on the office charge card and on the patient's receipt; the time and date for the next appointment is also given on the receipt. This system prevents error and confusion, and makes it easy to compile monthly reports of gross receipts.

It is also important to keep a running list of how many telephone inquiries have come in; their source; which individuals were evaluated; and, of these, what percentage became regular, weekly therapy patients. My average is about 60 percent, although an additional number were evaluated who did not need or elect to enter therapy. At the peak of my program, there were, on the average, one call or contact a day; at the low end, there were two or three a month. Keeping a close eye on these monthly figures helps you to cope with seasonal changes and lags, so you do not fall below your break-even point.

Follow-up on referrals is important to maintain your professional standing in the community, as well as to build your roster of clients. Referrals from physicians, psychologists, and social workers should have initial follow-up, or a copy of the evaluation report should be sent with the parent's knowledge and approval. Parents use their own discretion about sharing this information with the school system; some may fear the diagnostic label applied to their child might not be lifted after the problem has been properly treated. Other than these professional channels, which are already known and approved of by the family or the adult patient, information is never released verbally or in writing without written consent.

Legal Concerns/Insurance

A well-prepared therapist must also consider in advance what kind of information should be included in patients' files, in case of an unusual occurrence. As soon as possible after an emergency has occurred, the therapist should sit down (on that day, preferably) and note the time of the incident; what happened; who was involved; who saw it happen; and what action was taken and by whom. Also, if medical, fire, or police assistance was necessary, this should also be noted. You would want your report to be as complete and accurate as possible, and cosigned by a witness if possible. Such a "Report of Unusual Occurrence" could be very important, should you have to be defended in court for any subsequent legal action. Health professionals must be aware of the influence of large court settlements on attitudes in our society, and the increased likelihood of damage suits arising.

The possibility of law suits arising from the therapeutic situation leads to another important consideration, professional insurance. No one would expect to practice anywhere without professional liability insurance to cover their actions, or for any staff member that they employ. A good professional liability policy should provide coverage on the basis of incidents, no matter how long after you terminate your policy, should a claim be made against you. The group plan worked out by the AOTA and McGinnis and Associates, the endorsed Association carrier, provides such coverage.

As a therapist, you should carry insurance for yourself whether or not your place of employment does. In private practice, you should also carry personal property liability; if you practice in your own home, you should check out what kind of additional rider or policy you need beyond your homeowner's policy, because you have people on your premises who are paying for services.

What is often overlooked is the need for insurance to cover your overhead expenses if the mortgage, taxes for your facility, and business expenses depend on income from your own participation in your practice. You will need coverage of a disability overhead insurance policy to help meet the expenses of your practice should you become ill or be injured.

ORGANIZATION AND STRUCTURE OF THE PRACTICE

Case Load

In the military service, where I had set up the first program for the treatment of learning disorders for dependents of servicemen, I was responsible for treating more than forty children a week. The only way this could be accomplished was to treat them in groups, with parental assistance. There was sufficient homogeneity among the children to set up four groups, with some overlap of age allowing for advancement to the next group.

When I began my private practice, I started with individual therapy, with the hopes of grouping children as I had done before. This simply could not be done when working with small numbers of children. At that time, I averaged twelve children a week; this grew to about twenty-five to thirty children and adults. My experience has confirmed that a well-planned individual therapy session of fifty to sixty minutes has by far the greatest therapeutic impact; thirty minute sessions, except for the very young child, are too short. It would appear that one-hour sessions every other week would have greater impact than weekly sessions of half the time, which is customary in many school programs. Since we are striving to increase the child's attention span, we should not feed into the problem by offering hurried, brief sessions.

Evaluation

As those who are familiar with my text[4] will recall, I encourage both parents to attend the initial evaluation. For children under twelve years of age, the parent who brings the child usually attends the therapy sessions. Older children work with me alone; developments of the therapy session are shared with the parent at the end of the session.

There are advantages and disadvantages to parent observation. I believe I have provided the most effective therapy in this way, often giving the parent a rare opportunity to see the child perform in such a positive, productive manner. I feel at times I have given more therapy to the parent than to the child; at the very least, it makes for a more positive bond between them, which sometimes has hit a very low point prior to therapy.

The biggest disadvantage is that working in a triadic relationship such as this is emotionally draining for the therapist. In the last few years, it has at times become greater than I could manage in full days of seven or eight therapy sessions. Over the past year, I changed my policy; the parent sat in the waiting room, could overhear the general tone and content of what was transpiring, and then was filled in on details at the end of the session. Especially in cases where the emotional tension between parent and child is greatest, it was a relief as a therapist not to be under the added strain. The child may function better this way, but I lost some of the earlier benefits of reducing the negative impact of one on the other. In retrospect, I should perhaps have set a flexible policy which might, for some families, establish a parent-observation session every third or fourth meeting.

Since parents have been such an integral part of my program, it has been appropriate to establish and maintain a certain degree of formality in my professional interaction with them. I address them as "Mr." or "Mrs.," and I introduce myself as Miss Knickerbocker, which some of the young children shorten to "Bocker". I find that this style makes it easier to keep the focus of communication on therapy. If the child has a poor attention span, all efforts must be directed toward improving these skills. A breakdown in this type of formality promotes a "Chatty-Cathy" atmosphere.

During the last six years, I have had the opportunity to work with a number of high school and college students, as well as working adults. The contrast from working with young children has provided a new challenge. I've needed to change my techniques for this older age group. It has offered a much needed relief from the constant and draining emotional interaction required for successful results with a child.

As more adolescents and adults came into the program, I found that double, back-to-back sessions were more productive; the impact seemed greater by our concentrated effort over a longer period of time. Less time was lost to the opening and closing phases.

CLOSING A PRACTICE

When I was certain that I would be terminating my practice, I set a date, four months hence. From that point on, I only accepted new patients whom I felt could be treated within the four-month period. Patients already in therapy were told several months in advance of the termination date. Arrangements were made with another therapist who conducted a similar program, so that I could refer patients to her for continued or future needs. Unfortunately for some families, this would entail driving an ever greater distance.

To Sell or Not

I had made some attempts to sell my practice, and then decided against it. Since I would no longer be in the area, it would have been difficult for a new therapist to assume my caseload, referral base, and corporate name. No assurances of success could be offered. In order for such a sale to be beneficial to the new therapist and to the patients, I would have had to continue to work with both the patients and the new therapist to nurture and feed the therapeutic process.

There are ways to sell a practice, however, which had I been staying in the area, could have been considered. For instance, an agreed upon percentage of the annual gross receipts, averaged over the previous five years, could be used as one rule of thumb. The new therapist would pay, say, 40 percent of the five-year average gross receipts to the previous owner. Businesses are sold on such a basis. In addition to the patient load, the new therapist buys the good will, the contacts, the reputation, and the transfer of the corporate name, if there is one.

Closing Procedures

In pioneering the procedures for closing a private practice, I felt my professional responsibility to my patients had been fulfilled when I had notified active patients well in advance of the termination date, wrote to recent, but inactive, patients by mail, and provided each with the name and phone number of a member of my profession who could assist them.

Records of all patients I have treated for the entire eighteen years have been moved to my new location. Should anyone need the contents for further use or reference in a therapy program, they will be xeroxed. Only copies will be sent. In the event that any legal proceeding should ever arise, the complete and original record will be intact.

SUMMARY

This private practice, which I directed and conducted with some part-time assistance over the past eighteen years, was one of the first such full-time operations in the history of occupational therapy. Since there were no models to follow, I used my best professional training, my dedication to efficient and practical therapy procedures, and my experience in the military service with a parent-oriented program to establish my practice.

The most difficult aspect for me came in recognizing what knowledge of business would be helpful or even essential to the life of my practice. This I learned slowly, and not without making errors. I highly recommend that therapists involved in or contemplating a private practice should have some training in business skills; however, this should not be made an additional requirement for the basic occupational therapy curriculum.

Any business endeavor of the present day would be incomplete without computer services. Surely record keeping is made much more efficient. If I had had the availability of these hi-tech machines, I would have programmed them for in-depth documentation and research to compare, contrast, and improve treatment methods and techniques.

The critical issue of making a successful, self-supporting, independent practice is in knowing how to maintain an adequate cash flow; no matter how good a therapist you may be, you cannot provide therapy to those who need it unless you do it within a businesslike structure. The question is raised: "Can anyone make a go of it?" Like any other business operation, the answer lies in the difference between your gross receipts and your overhead. It is very hard to do. There are many variables which are often out of your control, especially in a children's program.

In the beginning, I used this rule of thumb: For every paid hour I worked per week, I expected to work one to two hours myself, or pay out in overhead for secretarial services, bookkeeping, clinical preparation, record keeping, cleaning, plus rent or the maintenance and upkeep of my building.

The stress on the therapist in private practice goes beyond merely financial problems. I have discussed some of the problems I faced in dealing with parents and children. I have also indicated the community outreach to other doctors, teachers, and local groups which can help you build and maintain your practice. The optimal length and structure of therapy sessions has also been addressed.

My experience is perhaps most unusual in that I decided to close my practice at the height of its success, when the patient load numbered twenty-five to thirty or more treatment hours per week. This timing was precipitated by a personal decision to move. However, I had decided long before that to close down before the end of the summer, so that I would have more time and opportunity to pursue other personal and professional interests. Because the closure came at a definite point, and was not a phased-out closing, the procedures that I followed were made more apparent, and may serve as a model for others to use.

CONCLUSION

I know of no other occupational therapy work that has a greater constellation of demands of physical, emotional, technical, and administrative skills—as well as personal maturity—than a private practice for learning-disordered children and adults. However, the rewards far exceed those of any other clinical setting or specialty area in which I worked over twenty years prior to the opening of my private practice. Today's therapists are far better prepared than I was to set out on such an endeavor. If they accept the risk and assume their full responsibilities, they can make a success of it.

NOTES

1. Princeton Center for Learning Disorders, 170 Cold Soil Road, Princeton, NJ 08540
2. *Private Practice,* Rockville, MD: American Occupational Therapy Association, Practice Division, 1982
3. *The Diagnostic and Statistical Manual of Mental Disorders,* 3d ed. Washington, DC: American Psychiatric Association, 1980, pp. 41–45
   The idenification numbers are as follows:
   314.00 Attention Deficit Disorder without Hyperactivity
   314.01 Attention Deficit Disorder with Hyperactivity
   314.80 Attention Deficit Disorder, Residual Type (adults)
4. Knickerbocker, BM: *A Holistic Approach to the Treatment of Learning Disorders,* Thorofare, NJ: Charles B. Slack, 1980

Developing Pediatric Programming in a Private Occupational Therapy Practice

Julie Shuer, MA, OTR
Laura Weiner, OTR

ABSTRACT. The purpose of this paper is to suggest to occupational therapists some introductory guidelines which might be followed in developing a private occupational therapy practice. Elements of a treatment program are discussed and examples drawn from a currently successful pediatric program which uses a sensory integrative approach in offering services.

Components of program development addressed in this paper include the purpose and content of screening as a recruitment device, how to structure an initial evaluation and parent conference, general treatment planning and goal setting, incorporating a theoretical frame of reference into practice, as well as clinic equipment in the private setting, documentation, discharge planning and finally, concepts of marketing for the beginning practice.

In recent years private practice has become an attractive and viable alternative for therapists wishing to leave traditional hospital settings. A growing number of occupational therapists have taken the opportunity to work in private practice with patients who are home based and with those in the

---

Julie Shuer is co-partner/developer of Occupational Therapy Services, a generalist occupational therapy practice at 5820 Wilshire Boulevard, Ste. 401, Los Angeles, California 90036.

Laura Weiner, currently completing requirements for a Master's degree in occupational therapy at the University of Southern California, is Director of Occupational Therapy at Santa Monica Hospital Medical Center in Santa Monica, California. She also provides pediatric therapy with Occupational Therapy Services in Los Angeles, and Hyland Clinic in Van Nuys, California.

This article appears jointly in *Private Practice in Occupational Therapy* (The Haworth Press, Inc., 1985), and *Occupational Therapy in Health Care*, Volume 2, Number 2 (Summer 1985).

53

well community also. Thereby they have expanded their horizons of personal and professional skills as well as increased their independence and flexibility. For one to venture into the private sector requires proficiency in a number of skills not generally addressed in an occupational therapy curriculum. Thus one must consider carefully such a move and plan well.

This paper focuses on the operation of a private practice in which there is pediatric programming which employs sensory integrative approaches in the treatment of children with learning disorders and developmental disabilities. The paper discusses a practice in which a specific theory is applied to a practice whose survival depends on its success as a business enterprise. The major components involved in such a program as addressed in this paper are: evaluation, treatment and marketing. However, related operational and planning activities also are discussed.

DEVELOPING CASELOAD

Program development first requires that one have an active caseload as well as opportunities for the continued recruitment of clients. Various opportunities for screening potential clients have been used successfully by the authors to develop a caseload. As a community service to private schools and pre-schools, occupational therapy screenings have been performed both as preventive services and to identify children who may have problems related to growth and development and learning potentials which are amenable to treatment. The twenty minute screenings are provided as a service to parents and to referral agencies and show whether indepth occupational therapy evaluations should be undertaken. Generally such screenings identify and differentiate appropriate evaluation candidates from those which are not suitable. Such screenings are a service which those potential referral agents may comfortably use since they do not involve additional expense to parents.

For this brief screening evaluation, clinical observations and parent/teacher reports may be sufficient or be used in conjunction with the Balcones Sensory Integration Test (BSIT) or the Quick Neurological Screening Test (QNST) (1, 2). The BSIT provides a base for evaluating brainstem and associated area responses in children ages six to nine years. Activities included in this tool are finger-nose-finger placement, heel toe walking, standing balance, testing with a dynamometer, checking tonic labyrinthine and asymmetrical tonic neck reflexes, ocular control, visual motor forms, arm postures, stereognosis and tactile graphics.[1] The QNST, appropriate for ages five through adult, assesses in gross terms maturity of motor development, skill in controlling large and small muscles, motor planning and sequencing, sense of rate of rhythm, spatial organization, visual and auditory perceptual skills, balance and disorders of attention.[2] Both the BSIT and the QNST can be used alone as screening tools or as components of a more comprehensive evaluation. Screening may also include the Southern California Postrotary Nystagmus Test (SCPNT).[3]

Experience in offering these screenings has yielded numerous appropriate referrals for treatment and continues to build visibility for the practice.

INITIATING TREATMENT

Initial Evaluations

When screening has indicated the need for further indepth evaluation, this is discussed with parents and an initial appointment is scheduled. Upon receipt of parental permission the referral source is notified and evaluation procedures are discussed. The purpose of the evaluation is twofold: (1) to define or diagnose a specific problem or its attributes, in one or more areas of behavior; and (2) to establish the baseline of a child's performance from which a treatment program can be developed and subsequent change measured.[4]

An initial evaluation of children ages four through ten usually includes the Southern California Sensory Integration Tests (SCSIT), and the Bruininks-Oseretsky Test of Motor Proficiency (BOTMP).[5,6] Children between the ages of two through five are evaluated using the Miller Assessment for Preschoolers (MAP).[7] Clinical observations are performed with all evaluations. Parents supplement the clinical evaluation by completing a Developmental History and an Activities of Daily Living Checklist.[8] It is recommended that the SCSIT, a series of 17 tests, requiring approximately 1-1/2 to 2 hours to administer, and the SCPNT be given by a certified examiner. These tools, to be used only for diagnostic purposes, assess areas of visual and somatosensory perception, motor performance and vestibular function.[3,5]

The BOTMP is composed of gross and fine motor subtests which includes running speed, balance, bilateral coordination, strength, upper limb coordination, response speed, visual motor control, and upper limb speed and dexterity. This test is appropriate for children ages four to fourteen and is useful both in diagnosis and in periodic re-evaluation.[6]

The MAP is intended to evaluate basic motor and sensory abilities, complex fine and oral motor abilities, cognitive language abilities, and cognitive abilities not requiring spoken language. Requiring only 20–30 minutes to administer, the test can be used either for screening or as a comprehensive clinical evaluative tool.[7]

The Developmental History yields information about birth history, motor milestones, self-care abilities, social/play behavior as well as perception including visual, tactile, vestibular, and auditory-language.[8] The Activities of Daily Living Checklist, completed by the parent or care giver, addresses mealtime activities, dressing, hygiene, bathing and toileting abilities, behavioral control and motivation, social interaction, independent play, postural muscle control, hand and visual perception activities, playground activities and communication.

For evaluating infants between two and thirty months of age the Bayley Scales of Infant Development are utilized for evaluative purposes.[9] This test is composed of both mental and motor scales and primarily assesses areas of sensory-perceptual acuities, perceptual awareness and discrimination, the acquisition of object constancy and memory, learning and problem solving abilities, degree of body control, coordination of the large muscles, and fine manipulatory skills of the hands and fingers.[9]

TREATMENT PLANNING

Parent Conference

A parent conference is scheduled as soon as the evaluation results have been analyzed in order to explain findings and needs and to plan for subsequent treatment. Preferably the child is not present, thus eliminating interruptions and the parents' or therapists' need to "censor" information or conversation. Initially the parents are provided with a typed copy of the evaluation report and test data and encouraged to read the information. Discussion is introduced with brief explanations of the evaluation tools describing what each test evaluates, how the tests were developed, and a brief synopsis of the tests reliability and validity. The child's performance during the evaluation, interpretation of the test results, a summary of the evaluation as well as implications for treatment and treatment recommendations are then discussed. From this process a treatment plan emerges.

It has been found helpful to parents to explain the underlying treatment philosophy and illustrate abstract concepts with graphs, charts and references. Frequently they are referred to Aryes' 1980 book entitled *Sensory Integration and the Child.*[10] To further illustrate concepts as used in practice, a tour of the treatment area is usually included.

To conclude the meeting, financial information is carefully discussed. Not only fee schedules and third party payment arrangements are covered but also therapists' availability in attending the child's educational planning meetings at the school. At this time also treatment schedules are presented and decided and intake information collected. Intake information should include the parents' home and work addresses and telephone numbers as well as the name, address and telephone numbers of the physician of the family or of the child.

In concluding, be sure to set aside several minutes to clarify issues and answer any questions which the parent may have. However, feel free to set a time limit on such discussions and to draw the meeting courteously to a close. Encourage the parents to call with any further questions, but suggest the hours you are available for such calls.

It may be helpful to provide material in writing to be reviewed at home since parent conferences incorporate an ex-
tensive amount of information and may be difficult for the
parent to listen to, comprehend and accept. Such literature
might include copies of the typed evaluation report, fee
schedules, treatment schedules and reference material about
the treatment program to be undertaken. Again, encourage
the parents to call if they have questions since parent cooperation is so critical to treatment success.

Objectives and Treatment Plans

Once determined that treatment will be initiated, goals,
objectives and specific treatment plans need to be established.
Plans for treatment are developed individually, consistent
with each child's needs, based on the long and short term
goals which are established following evaluation.

Overall long term goal may be stated generally perhaps in
terms of the theoretical concepts of treatment being used. In
a setting where a sensory integrative approach to treatment is
followed, a long term goal might be phrased as:

> Long term goal: to improve Johnny's ability to organ-
> ize his behavior in an appropriate manner in interaction
> with his surroundings.

Achievement of such long term goals is determined by progress in activity directed to several short term goals and objectives and phrased as:

> Long term goal: to improve organization of behavior.
> Short term goal: to increase child's ability to attend to
> a task.
> Objective: the child will be able to attend to at least
> one task for 20 minutes during each treatment session.

Records of clinical observation and re-administration of tests
serve to measure specific gains from treatment.

Objectives set goals in motion by providing a structural
basis for treatment. Because a therapists' understanding of
the theoretical concepts underlying treatment affect not only

goal setting but specific treatment activities and plans, considerations for applying concepts of treatment are now addressed.

Concepts of Treatment

In order to provide quality treatment it is important to apply a frame of reference to treatment plans, one that incorporates concepts pertinent to the client's needs. In the experience of the authors treating a great number of children, it appears that knowledge and application of a sensory integrative approach is not only helpful but essential. For the purpose of this paper the following definition applies: sensory integrative therapy is designed to provide activities that give stimulation to a child in accordance with his neurological needs so as to elicit adaptive responses. The focus of therapy is to provide vestibular, proprioceptive and tactile stimulation. Treatment usually incorporates full body movement on specialized equipment and does not focus on teaching discrete skills. Therapy is provided by a skilled therapist in a specialized structured environment which enables the child to direct his own activities. The ultimate goal of therapy is to improve the child's sensory integrative processes. Therapeutic effects will appear in the increased ability of the child to direct his own activity and meet environmental demands.[10,11,12]

To illustrate the application of the sensory integrative approach used in the authors' practice, a set of treatment principles extracted from the literature highlights and clarifies important sensory integrative concepts which can be helpful in developing a treatment program in which the patient and parent are integrated and oriented in an orderly manner. Although not an exhaustive list, it is designed to be used by experienced therapists wishing to use sensory integrative treatment.[13]

1. Treatment is guided by the therapist's interpretation of the child's performance on the SCSIT, clinical observation and other evaluations.
2. Treatment is provided on a one-therapist-to-one-child basis.

3. The child in therapy is self-directed within the structure set by the therapist.
4. Activities are adapted in accordance with the child's response in treatment.
5. Sensory integrative therapy does not teach specific skills nor tasks but rather enhances organization of adapted responses. In that way outcomes of therapy are more generalizable.
6. Physical movement in therapy focuses on sensorimotor function and usually involves full body movement.
7. A limited amount of equipment designed to meet specific neurological needs of the child is presented.
8. The type and amount of sensory stimulation the child receives should be monitored carefully.
9. The therapist evaluates the child's response to therapy. This involves comparing the child's elicited responses to pre-therapy test scores, reviewing the written progress notes on the child's performance, discussions with parents and teachers regarding the child's behavior, and his academic performance.
10. The effects of therapy take time and will not be seen immediately. Studies suggest therapy programs should be at least 2 hours weekly for 6 months, but this varies depending on the child's needs.

In summary, using a frame of reference such as sensory integration which incorporates specific concepts and treatment sequences along with goals that are practical and strategies possible to measure, a therapist can develop a useful treatment program.

EQUIPMENT AND OTHER PRACTICE REQUIREMENTS

The discussion to follow is limited to planning in a pediatric practice such as the one described above. Thus, all details may not apply to other settings, even though basic principles will.

Equipment

In order to determine equipment needs in a private pediatric practice by way of equipment and other operational requirements, one must look at the treatment approach you plan to follow. For example, the major focus of the sensory integrative treatment approaches is to provide clients with activities involving vestibular stimulation. In a relatively small space these can be easily provided through the use of equipment suspended from a sturdy beam in an A-frame structure. Constructed of redwood, the top of the A-frame is reinforced by steel bracing, the cross brace is also well reinforced. Eyebolts placed equidistant across the length of the beam provide places for the attachment of swivel hooks with carabiners from which various equipment is suspended (and easily detached). If more length is required, a heavy soldered chain can be added to lower items nearer to the floor.

Many different pieces of equipment are used with the A-frame structure, providing various types of sensory input and opportunities to elicit a variety of adaptive responses. Equipment used should vary not only in amount and type of sensory input provided but also in terms of the complexity and level of interaction required. Regardless of the amount of space available the following types of equipment are essential to a fully equipped occupational therapy clinic providing sensory integrative treatment. These include, but are not limited to: hammock-type net, inner tubes of various sizes, bolster swing, platform swing, a carpeted barrel, tiltboards, a scooterboard, a ramp, trampoline, Bobath ball, trapeze, bolsters, a T-stool, climbing equipment, and a variety of tactile stimulating items such as brushes, blankets, textured cloths, bubble ball bath and crazy foam. Eye-hand coordination items such as foam/fleece balls, target games and bean bags are also handy as are pulleys, cuff weights and weighted vests.[11]

Safety

Regardless of the treatment approaches that one uses in a private practice setting the client's safety is foremost in planning and equipping a treatment area. Because of this the following precautions have been taken in the authors' program: mats are placed under the patient whenever and wherever there is a possibility that he might fall; all equipment is put away after use to leave the treatment area uncluttered; small equipment should have a storage place and be kept there when not in use, and not on the floor; vibrators, hard brushes and other small items of treatment in the authors' clinic are kept in small boxes in a cabinet nearby; equipment that will hang on pegs or hooks should be hung there as soon after its use as is convenient.

In addition the use of suspended equipment can be hazardous. For example, when having a child swing prone in a net or hammock one must be sure the child keeps his head up to avoid neck injury; when having him do somersaults be sure he tucks his head down and under. A therapist's ability to maintain an organized treatment area not only provides a safer environment but is less distracting and thereby helps the client to be more organized. Also, having the child assist with clean up helps him organize himself in completing the session and assists the therapist in preparing for the next client.

In case of emergencies a First Aid kit and an instant cold pack should be kept close by in the treatment area. Also it is ideal to have a telephone in the actual treatment area for the safety of all. Finally, because of all the potentials for problems related to treatment, it is essential that both the corporation/operator of the practice and each individual therapist carry professional liability insurance with maximum coverage. This is readily available from McGinnis and Associates, the AOTA recognized vendor. Certification in cardiopulmonary resuscitation (CPR) should also be a requirement for all treating clinicians.

Documentation

Clear accurate records of treatment are essential in any program. Each clinic obviously develops systems to meet its needs. Nonetheless certain guiding principles pertain for documentation regardless of the setting. It is important to document positive and negative aspects of each treatment session as well as overall progress, regression or lack of progress in treatment.

Daily notes summarize each treatment session and might be written in one of the following ways:

1. A narrative format.
2. A narrative format which is highlighted in the margins. The highlighting is to alert the reader/therapist to spe-

cific areas of interest and is helpful in reviewing daily notes when writing formal progress reports. Examples of highlighting may include: praxis, sensory processing, organization of behavior, social and emotional behaviors and communication.

3. The Subjective, Objective, Assessment, Plan (SOAP) note format.

Daily treatment notes as well as formal re-evaluations are legal medical records and must be dated with time noted and signed by a registered occupational therapist. Later, these daily treatment notes are synthesized to contribute to the documentation of re-evaluation. In addition, informal reports from parents as well as formal and informal reports from physicians and teachers should be part of the record and must be documented when they too contribute to the re-evaluation report.

Formal re-evaluation and/or interim progress reports should be timed according to contractual agreements, insurance policies, requirements of third party payors and parent needs and requests. Re-evaluation should involve use of the same tools as used in initial evaluation in order to assess progress validly. The formal re-evaluation report should, of course, be dated and should contain basic information: the child's name, birthdate, date of first treatment, parents' names, address and phone number, referral source, treatment frequency, and presenting problems. If available, pre- and post-therapy test scores, parent and teacher reports, as well as a summary of clinical observations should be noted. Daily treatment notes are synthesized and specific, measurable, dated incidents from the treatment notes reflecting changes are included. For example:

> Sue is currently able to maintain attention to task for a 20 minute period as charted on 3-10-83 and 2-7-83. This is compared to her prior limited attention span of five minutes as indicated in progress notes of 5-7-82. She is more alert and aware as demonstrated by her increased desire to initiate active exploration of the environment.

Comments as well as discussion regarding the re-evaluation, along with a general summary and overall impressions and recommendations should be provided. Long term and short term goals and objectives are re-stated with appropriate adjustments based on current status.

A typed copy of the formal re-evaluation should be provided to the parents with discussion in a formal parent conference. Copies of the re-evaluation report should be sent to the referral source (as appropriate), to the physician and, with parental permission only, to the teacher and any other involved team member.

Termination of Treatment

During the course of treatment it is appropriate to look ahead to termination and continually re-evaluate progress. Is this child achieving the goals and objectives established in this program? Have the goals and objectives already been achieved or are they still appropriate? If not, what can I, as the therapist, be doing to facilitate this process? Frequent consideration of these and other questions related to progress may help to guide discharge planning.

The actual discharge process is usually initiated following formal re-evaluation and is generally based on one of the following outcomes: (1) the child may not have shown significant progress during treatment as evidenced from clinical observation, formal evaluation and/or parent and teacher reports, or (2) the child has achieved the long term goals and objectives (or most of them) established within the treatment program.

It is important to consider that in either circumstance discontinuing treatment sessions may be a difficult issue for both parent and child. To ease the termination, discharge needs to be well planned and executed. While the period until discharge will vary with each individual child, when possible it is helpful to gradually reduce the number and frequency of treatment sessions. For example, approximately two months prior to discharge let the child and parents know that the child has performed well and will soon no longer need to come to treatment sessions. If the child is being seen twice weekly, cut back to once a week for a month. Continue to evaluate the child's progress and assess how well he is performing both in treatment and at home and in school. The program can be further tapered to one visit every two weeks or one time a month for one or two visits until treatment is finally ended.

At the end let the child and the parent know that they are welcome to come back to the clinic and visit and assure the parent of your availability should questions arise. Encourage the parent to feel free to contact you, that you too are interested in their child's continued progress. In cases where the child has not progressed, attempt to provide the parents with alternative assistance through other community resources.

MARKETING

As was indicated earlier, the survival of any community based occupational therapy practice is dependent on an active caseload. This is developed through continual and consistent promotional efforts. Therefore one should explore many ways of promoting or marketing one's practice. Promotional activities directed toward your particular target audience may include offering cost-free screenings (as previously described), advertising (the kind depend on your resources and the results achieved), publicity in local and specialty publications, and personal contact with potential referral sources. Paid advertising, as in a specialty newspaper, is costly and reaches a large population, but may not produce referrals in proportion with its cost. For example advertisements in *L.A. Parent Magazine* are placed by pediatricians, allied health professionals, special educators and private schools. Free publicity, often the most productive, may also be acquired through press releases of events in which you participated or by actual face-to-face contact in community services programs such as in health fairs.

Personal contact remains as the best avenue for promoting one's service. Developing relationships with your client's physician, teacher or speech/language pathologist allows one the opportunity not only to talk about the child who is your client, but also offers the chance to "sell" your services and the benefits of occupational therapy. Doing complimentary screenings at preschools has been discussed. However, offering to teach inservice sessions to teachers or networking with other allied health professionals and occupational therapists in the area for referrals are other important means for helping your practice grow.

Even though once established, it is important to continue by participation in continuing education and conferences, providing monthly inservicing for staffs in referral agencies and developing clinical research activities. It is not enough to just do a good job of professional practice when in a private practice. In order to grow personally and for occupational therapy as a profession to grow, therapists must communicate with professional collegues via professional journals, generic publications and professional organizations, as well as continually re-evaluating one's effectiveness. Reviewing service demand, kinds of referrals, trends in health care delivery as well as client satisfaction on a regular basis provides information that guides future growth activity in a private practice.

SUMMARY

This paper has discussed a private practice pediatric occupational therapy program in which a sensory integrative approach is used as a basis for programming. The purpose was to provide some guidelines to others considering private practice. Basic information included can be generalized for serving clients with different needs using different treatment approaches in other settings. The paper discussed several key components some of which were specific to a pediatric treatment program. These components included screening, initial evaluation and baseline data, parent consultation, treatment planning and goal setting, application of concepts of treatment, equipment, space and other operating requirements, documentation and discharge planning. A brief discussion of marketing a pediatric occupational therapy practice concluded the paper.

To develop a well integrated pediatric practice requires that client and parent be oriented in a consistent and orderly manner to the goals and activities of the program. In a practice setting one can do this unusually well if one plans each of the key components of the treatment relationship well.

REFERENCES

1. Jones C & Monkhouse M, *Balcones Sensory Integration Screening,* Texas Occupational Therapy Association, 1981

2. Mutti M, Sterling HM, & Spalding NV, *Quick Neurological Screening Test,* Novato, CA: Academic Therapy Publications, 1978

3. Ayres AJ, *Southern California Postrotary Nystagmus Test,* Los Angeles: Western Pschological Services, 1980

4. Banus, BS, *The Developmental Therapist,* Thorofare, NJ: Charles B Slack, Inc, 1971

5. Ayres AJ, *Southern California Sensory Integration Tests Revised 1980,* Los Angeles: Western Psychological Services, 1980

6. Bruininks RH, *Bruininks-Oseretsky Test of Motor Proficiency,* Circle Press, Minn: American Guidance Service, 1978

7. Miller LJ, *Miller Assessment for Preschoolers,* Littleton, CO: The Foundation for Knowledge in Development, 1982

8. Ayres AJ, *Developmental History,* Unpublished manuscript

9. Bayley N, *Bayley Scales of Infant Development,* New York: The Psychological Corporation, 1969

10. Ayres AJ, *Sensory Integration and the Child,* Los Angeles: Western Psychological Services, 1980

11. Ayres AJ, *Sensory Integration and Learning Disorders.* Los Angeles: Western Psychological Services, 1972

12. Ayres AJ, Learning disabilities and the vestibular system, *Journal of Learning Disabilities* 1978, *11,* page 30–40

13. Weiner LB, *Utilization of the Sensory Integrative Treatment Approach Within the Pediatric Population,* Unpublished Master's thesis, University of California, Los Angeles 1983

The Airplane:
Another Solution to Transportation
in a Rural Private Practice

James R. Christen, OTR

ABSTRACT. As a rural private practice in occupational therapy expanded to meet the service requests in a large, sparsely populated area, the need for fast, efficient transportation became obvious. A private pilot's license was acquired and then an airplane was purchased to meet that transportation need. The private practice, geographical area and the intervention methods are reviewed. The efficiency, cost, safety and practicality of flying, and its effect on the success of the private practice are then described.

An individual practice[1] was started in the geographical center of Nebraska (located in the town of Broken Bow—population 4,000) in 1976, following a subjective analysis of the possible needs for occupational therapy services.

THE GEOGRAPHICAL AREA

The 1980 census lists Nebraska's population as 1.6 million—this total is less than many of the nation's metropolitan areas. With an area of 77,227 square miles (475 miles long, 200 miles wide) the state's population density is 20.7. However, approximately two-thirds of the population is concentrated in the eastern one-sixth of the state, so the population

James R. Christen is owner/operator of a private practice in occupational therapy with headquarters in Broken Bow, Nebraska. Because of scarcity of therapists in rural areas of the state, his caseload is spread over a wide geographic area and covers many kinds of patients.

This article appears jointly in *Private Practice in Occupational Therapy* (The Haworth Press, Inc., 1985), and *Occupational Therapy in Health Care*, Volume 2, Number 2 (Summer 1985).

69

density of the greater portion of the state is closer to 6 people per square mile and less than that in many areas. The American Heritage Dictionary defines rural as applying to sparsely settled or agricultural country as distinct from settled communities,[2] so it can be safely said that this is a rural practice. With the area being sparsely populated it does have some of the "strong flavor of Appalachia"[3] and some of the abject conditions described by Seig.[4] However, the area has no more of a monopoly on poverty and ignorance than it does on wealth and intelligence. There are many area farmers, ranchers and businessmen whose assets easily exceed the one million dollar mark. (As an example, Hyannis, a ranching community town of 330 in west central Nebraska has historically had the honor of having the greatest number of millionaires per capita in the state.) Several native businessmen, physicians, psychologists, etc., are nationally and internationally known and involved. This area being my home, my bias is understood.

Health care services and facilities are limited in many areas and it is not uncommon for people to travel up to 100 miles to obtain services. In contrast "Nebraska ranks second among the states in the number of licensed nursing-home beds in relation to its elderly population, according to the General Accounting Office."[5] Although the people accept these facts as part of living in the area, the pioneering spirit is still strong and efforts are being made to improve the conditions. Thus the area was found to be receptive to the possible benefits of occupational therapy, and as Devereaux suggested,[3] the teaching/training by an occupational therapist enhances the effectiveness of the total treatment process and in turn, facilitates more referrals.

THE PRIVATE PRACTICE

The caseload of the "Practice" is difficult to define, particularly in terms of "caseload" as it refers to the number of patients being treated by a therapist in an occupational therapy department. The "Practice" consists of agreements/contracts with various agencies, facilities and individuals with each of these entities having a "caseload" in the classical sense. The variety of agencies, facilities and individuals is such that the occupational therapist must serve as a "generalist".

In pediatrics, the "Practice" provides service to the State Department of Social Services/Services for Crippled Children's (SCC) program. This consists of serving on the monthly OT/PT Diagnostic Treatment Planning and Cerebral Palsy Clinics in four area cities located from 65 to 105 road miles from the home office. The SCC clinics recommend the amount of OT/PT services to be provided to the pediatric population, with the services then provided in, and reimbursed by, the local school district/State Department of Education. Services are provided in approximately fifteen school districts, located up to 135 road miles away from my office.

In geriatrics, the "Practice" has provider agreements with thirteen nursing homes (ICF & SNF), with the most distant being 225 road miles away. Agreements with four hospitals and a Home Health Agency (physical disabilities) could involve travel up to 70 road miles. On a weekly basis, psychiatric occupational therapy services are provided 105 road miles away to a state regional psychiatric hospital.

One of the more unusual provisions of occupational therapy services that the "Practice" has enjoyed, has been the request from two lawyers to provide evaluations/reports on their clients for Social Security Disability Court appeals when the report of the occupational therapy evaluation became the determining factor in the cases.

This total caseload is spread over a monthly to quarterly schedule, and visits to facilities are often combined. Frequently, the schedule is arranged so that travel in an area will include stops in two or more places. For example: the SCC Clinics usually end in the early afternoon, so the remainder of the afternoon is then scheduled for school visits, individual patients, etc., in that city or perhaps a Home Health patient visit on the way back to Broken Bow.

In addition to serving as a "generalist" the occupational therapist is functioning primarily in a "consultant" role, as described by Mazer.[6] The majority of the intervention time is spent working with the staff (or parents in pediatric cases). This involves working through the facility's system of treatment; i.e., the Individual Educational Plan in schools, the Overall Plan of Care in nursing homes, the Comprehensive Treatment Plan in the psychiatric hospital and the Individual Program Plan in the ICF-MR unit. Staff inservice presentations are also used as a means of affecting change in patient treatment.

The preceding description of the "Practice" and the geographical area that it covers further underscores, as documented by others,[4,7] the need for unique transportation when providing services in a rural area.

TRANSPORTATION MODES

The automobile is a common mode of transportation and serves the purpose well in the rural area. One very seldom encounters anything resembling a traffic jam (although I have had to wait up to five minutes, a few times, for a farmer transporting a large piece of equipment or a rancher moving cattle along or across a highway). The transportation problem can also be considered as a "time" problem, with "time" being an allocatable resource. One hour of traveling time by automobile, in this area, transports one approximately 50 road miles.

In December 1976, with the "Practice" just getting started, an opportunity arose to sign a provider agreement with a nursing home 135 road miles away. The nursing home was establishing an ICF-MR unit and anticipated needing occupational therapy services on a quarterly basis. The approximately three hours of travel time (six hours round trip), on a quarterly basis, was not felt to be unreasonable as the "Practice" needed the business. However, the need for occupational therapy service rapidly increased and by July of 1977, weekly visits were being made. The amount of time spent traveling had become unreasonable. In analyzing the situation, three options were considered: (a) terminate the agreement, (b) move to a location closer to the facility, (c) use a different mode of transportation—flying. The first option was felt to be unacceptable, as the "Practice" was still struggling to get established and the business was welcomed. The second option was also rejected as the geographically centered location of the "Practice" was proving beneficial in developing other agreements for services. The third option could not only solve the existing problem, but provide a means of developing more business and, at the same time, actualize a childhood dream. The decision was made to acquire a private pilot's license.

It was already known that the Broken Bow Municipal Airport offered flight instructions and aircraft rental, so a visit was made to the airport to obtain the particular details. After explaining the plan to my banker and obtaining a loan, ground school and flight instructions were started in the fall of 1977, and the private pilot's license was received in March of 1978.

The Dictionary of Occupational Titles[8] worker functions rating for an airplane pilot is .263 as compared to .121 for an occupational therapist. The worker function ratings are a range from simple (higher numbers) to complex (0) with each rating including those that are simpler and excluding the more complex. Thus, an airplane pilot at .263 is said to react to Data at the Analyzing level, People at the Speaking-Serving level, and Things at the Driving-Operating level. An occupational therapist is said to react to Data at the Coordinating level, People at the Instructing level and Things at the Precision Working level. Therefore, according to this reference, there should be no problem with an occupational therapist becoming an airplane pilot.

Parts 61 and 67 of the Federal Aviation Regulations[9] list the requirements for a private pilot's certificate. Generally stated, this involves obtaining a medical certificate, passing a written exam, having at least 20 hours of flight instruction and 20 hours of solo flight and passing a flight test. Another 40 hours of training, passing another written exam and another flight test are required to obtain an instrument rating. Part 91 of the Federal Aviation Regulations gives the requirements for Visual Flight Rules (VFR) and Instrument Flight Rules (IFR). For VFR flying, the pilot must maintain a required amount of visibility and distance from clouds, whereas IFR allows the pilot to fly in clouds—guided by instruments in the airplane, on the ground, and contact with an instrument flight control center.

EFFICIENCY

How efficient is private flying? The primary savings is time. In a sample analysis of one month's flying, 20 hours were flown traveling approximately 2,600 miles. Traveling to the same places by road would have resulted in 3,000 miles, and 60 hours of travel time (at an average of 50 mph). Thus, a savings of 40 hours was realized. The value of those 40 hours could be calculated by multiplying it by the "Practice"s' hourly rate; however, those were 40 hours that the "Practice" would not otherwise have had available in which to provide services so it is felt that the benefits are greater than what simple multiplication would indicate. Perhaps a more precise formula would be: value equals time saved multiplied by the hourly rate plus the benefits of the services provided, or $V = (T \times R) + B$. However, the benefits of the service provided are difficult to assign a numerical value to as they include both the facility's or patient's direct benefits and the benefits to the "Practice" in increased exposure that can result in more referrals.

It is also possible that this monthly time savings could be regarded as a one-fourth full-time-equivalent employee. To cite another example: Monthly visits to a nursing home 135 road miles away are combined with visits to a school 123 road miles from Broken Bow. The nursing home and school are 40 road miles apart, for a total round-trip mileage of 298 miles (5.98 hours travel time at 50 mph). By air, the round-trip mileage is 224 miles and the travel time 1.75 hours. This generates a savings, in one day, of approximately 4 hours; i.e., a one-half full-time-equivalent employee.

COST

An aviation rule-of-thumb is that over 150-200 hours of flying per year justifies owning a plane instead of renting one. Owning a plane also provides a marked degree of scheduling flexibility over renting. These factors were considered when the decision was made to purchase a plane in August of 1978, as airplanes had been rented for use up to that time. The

"Practice"s' current aircraft, a 1978 Cessna Model 172N was purchased in March of 1979 with a 10-1/2 percent bank loan. The normal business tax advantages (investment credit, depreciation, etc.) further reduce the "apparent" cost so that when the travel time savings is considered (at a simple multiplication rate) the "Practice"s' flying cost is comparable to driving cost. The determining factor between flying or driving is the time saved. In this geographical area, with the distances traveled, the "Practice"s' current airplane is efficient. If one were regularly flying greater distances, or from an area of significantly higher elevation, different types of aircraft could be more appropriate.

SAFETY

In spite of the "front page" publicity that airplane crashes receive, private flying is safe. 91.1 percent of the 1982 transportation fatalities were highway related, while only 3.2 percent were aviation related.[10] Even on long cross-country flights, other aircraft are seldom seen as regulations require pilots to fly at certain altitudes depending on the direction of flight—there are "highways" in the sky.

Airplanes do have their limitations and these must be respected. Each airplane has a maximum gross weight that includes the fuel, passengers and baggage. The pilot can vary the amount of fuel or load to meet a particular flight's requirements as long as the maximum gross weight is not exceeded. Each type of aircraft has its takeoff and landing capabilities, though modified by: the load being carried, the air temperature, the airport elevation, the type of runway surface and the wind velocity. The pilot does not always need a long, hard surfaced runway—landings and takeoffs are possible (and have been made) from farm fields.

The pilot's limitations must also be respected and accepted. A VFR rated pilot needs to avoid IFR conditions. Spatial disorientation, to the point of not even knowing which way is up, is possible. The training for IFR flying teaches the pilot to trust the airplane's instruments and ignore the body's vestibular system.

PRACTICALITY

A potential problem with flying is arranging for ground transportation once you arrive at the destination airport. Surprisingly, this is seldom a problem. The agreements/contracts are made with the understanding that I will be flying and that ground transportation will need to be provided by the facility. In most cases, the airports have a Fixed Base Operator (FBO) that can be called via the aircraft's communication radio while one is still ten to fifteen minutes away. The FBO staff then telephones the facility and advises them of my impending arrival (i.e., requesting transportation). Also, the FBOs usually have one or more "courtesy cars" that can be "borrowed" and for which one leaves a small "donation" upon returning. In the larger cities, the FBOs have rental cars or city taxis are available. When flying to an airport that does not have a FBO, I use a telephone in my airplane hanger to call the facility just before taking off, and give an estimate of my arrival time.

Weather can be a serious problem. It is standard procedure to check both the existing conditions and the forecast for the expected time of the return trip (this is done through the Federal Aviation Administration's Flight Service Stations). There have been times when it was possible/safe to fly but not drive; e.g., shortly after a winter storm when the sky was perfectly clear, the airports had been opened but some of the roads were still closed. More frequently, inclement weather forces the cancelation of flying plans and it is still possible/safe to drive. Dense fog, blizzards, etc., present conditions in which it is not possible/safe to fly or drive. Again, agreements/contracts are made with the understanding that weather conditions can, and do, affect the ability to travel. When travel is not possible, the visit is canceled and rescheduled. In such cases, a visit to a closer facility is substituted, if possible, or the time is spent in the home office (doing paperwork or reading).

In spite of weather problems the airplane has been a practical mode of transportation. There are more referrals than the "Practice" can accommodate. Time saving office procedures (e.g., using dictation and a typist, having a bookkeeper, etc.) are utilized. The consultation intervention role[6] is effective in reaching a larger number of patients. Referrals are made to other occupational therapists whenever possible.

IN CONCLUSION

Using an airplane for transportation by a therapist in a rural occupational therapy practice will not be feasible in many settings; however, in this particular "Practice" it does work. In fact, it has worked too well! The benefits of occupational therapy services are being recognized in this rural area of Nebraska and consequently more services are being requested than the "Practice" is able to meet.

Rural areas have liabilities for living and working just as urban areas do. Perhaps if more attention (including during professional education) were given to the needs and rewards of practice in rural areas, then more therapists would consider and undertake rural practice. Rural health care service needs are tremendous, the challenges formidable yet manageable, and the rewards . . . isn't this what ocupational therapy is supposed to be?

REFERENCES

1. Frazian BJ: Establishing and administering a private practice in a hospital setting. *Am J Occup Ther* 32: 296–300, 1978

2. *American Heritage Dictionary,* Second College Edition, Boston: Houghton Mifflin Company 1982, p 1079

3. Devereaux, EB: Community home health care in the rural setting. In *Willard and Spackman's Occupational Therapy,* HL Hopkins, HD Smith, Editors, Philadelphia: JB Lippincott Co 653-671, 1978

4. Sieg KW: Rural health and the role of occupational therapy. *Am J Occup Ther* 29: 75–80, 1975

5. *Omaha World Herald,* 17 January 1984

6. Mazer, JL: The Occupational Therapist as Consultant. *Am J Occup Ther* 23: 417–421, 1969

7. Magrun WM, Tigges KN: A transdisciplinary mobile intervention program for rural areas. *Am J Occup Ther* 36: 90–94, 1982

8. *Dictionary of Occupational Titles,* Fourth Edition. Washington, D.C.: US Government Printing Office 1977, pp 59 146; 1369–1371

9. Colvin JK, Ed: *AOPA's Handbook for Pilots 1983.* Bethesda: Aircraft Owners and Pilots Association, 1983, pp 271–408

10. "1984 Aviation Fact Card", *AOPA Newsletter,* January 1984, p 8

Occupational Therapists as Publishers and Trainers in the Field of Aging

Elizabeth S. Deichman, EdM, OTR
Mary V. Kirchhofer, BS, OTR

ABSTRACT. This is an account of how two occupational therapists, specialists in the field of aging, formed a publishing company to disseminate their ideas in an effort to help change attitudes about aging. The paper touches briefly on the organization, financing and staffing, the acquisition of manuscripts and materials, and how distribution by mail order was developed. Further there are descriptions of the development of workshops, inservice training activities and audio-visual materials. The authors show how community outreach has led to the expansion of their business into unforeseen areas including work with children of aging parents, intergenerational groups and a public school curriculum.

In the '60s and '70s there was little interest shown by medical professionals, including occupational therapists, in the field of aging. Those who did become involved did so because they had as their philosophy that "living is for everyone." This is the reason the authors became more and more deeply involved. For many years they were actively involved in clinical practice, teaching, writing, pursuing grants and working with programs in the community in the field of aging.

As a result of their work as consultants to activity directors particularly, they saw daily the need to help the often minimally trained workers in nursing facilities to develop effective

Elizabeth S. Deichman is President and Mary V. Kirchhofer is Vice President of Potentials Development for Health and Aging Services, Inc., 775 Main Street, Suite 325, Buffalo, NY 14203.

This article appears jointly in *Private Practice in Occupational Therapy* (The Haworth Press, Inc., 1985), and *Occupational Therapy in Health Care*, Volume 2, Number 2 (Summer 1985).

79

programs. At all levels of personnel there was a lack of understanding that aging imposes no limit on the needs for love, respect, valid roles, meaningful activity, freedom of choices and that when these needs are not filled, health suffers. The growth of the nation's health movement has brought to awareness the close relationships between mental, emotional and physical health. This has always been a basic tenet of occupational therapy philosophy, but somehow it had been ignored in work with the elderly.

THE EVOLUTION OF A BUSINESS VENTURE

In time, as some shocking stories about nursing home care began to influence federal and state governments, funds became available for improving the quality of that care. As a result, in 1969 the Occupational Therapy Department at the State University of New York at Buffalo (SUNYAB) was designated to institute training courses for persons involved in work with the aged in western New York. One of the authors (Deichman) planned and implemented a course, via two-way radio, which formed a part of the tele-lecture series operated by the Lake Area Regional Medical Program.

This later led to the first 64 hour training course for activity directors in Buffalo in the Spring of 1971, and subsequently to similar courses in Syracuse and in Erie, Pennsylvania. The presentations by the variety of professionals involved were taped by the author who edited and assembled them in the form of a book published by Lakes Area Health Education Center. At a later date the rights to the book were acquired by the author who, with others, edited and enlarged it. In 1975 DOK,[1] a local publisher in Buffalo which specializes in materials for gifted and talented young people, agreed to publish *Working with the Elderly*[2] on a shared cost basis. This success inspired the author to consider developing and publishing more training materials as there was obvious need.

In the meantime author #2 (Kirchhofer) started an adult day care center with Area Agency on Aging (AAA) funds and was also directing a seniors' center financed with block grant funds. She too saw the enormous needs among practitioners providing direct service to elders. Together the two therapists decided to become business women in earnest.

Potentials Development

What resulted was Potentials Development, a publishing company and the business venture to be described. Once the decision was made, next came any number of problems to be solved, principal among them locating materials developed/ written by experienced and innovative workers in the field of aging. The need was for practical, original educational materials, couched in non-academic language. A search of the local area produced some good results. Three projects actually launched the business: (1) an activity director who used a series of interesting "quizzes" to facilitate conversations among nursing home residents agreed to prepare and submit them for publication; (2) DOK passed along a manuscript on wheelchair dancing they had received as a result of being the publisher of *Working with the Elderly;* (3) a compilation of an audio-visual resource catalogue[3] already begun seemed ripe for publication. These three projects together with the distribution of *Working with the Elderly,* for which there was increasing demand, formed the nucleus of this emerging business.

Organizing for Business

The authors readily recognized that they knew little about running a business. Accordingly several steps were taken to fill their needs. First, a lawyer was consulted to help with the official organizing, deciding on profit or non-profit status. The decision was made to be a for-profit or tax paying proprietary company, though with hindsight, this may have proven an error of judgement since grants could not be sought and mailing costs were much higher, a considerable expense in a mail-order business. This proved especially true for this company which grew tremendously within two years.

Second, one of the "partners" took a short course in how to start a small business. This, while helpful in some ways, served to raise almost as many questions as it solved.

Examples of some of the decisions that had to be made following registration as a business with both city and county were:

1. Choosing a location from which to operate which would be affordable, and deciding on an official address for

post office purposes. One of the authors' homes was chosen initially, for which she could take tax deduction.
2. Raising necessary capital to begin, acquire equipment, pay staff and establish credit. One author invested the funds, the other did all editoral and office work at the beginning.
3. Raising further development funds. To do this, firms listed in the proposed resource catalogue were contacted seeking contributions to cover the cost of printing. This strategy produced some additional funds.
4. Acquiring equipment and staff to produce initial materials. Local part-time persons (typist and graphic artist) were hired and they, with the partners, produced camera-ready materials for the local printer.
5. Marketing strategies. Both mail order and advertising journals were considered. Advertising was expensive and the response to a few trials was poor. Mail order, therefore, was given priority. Mailing labels of local, regional and national aging facilities were purchased, and a bulk mailing permit secured. A mailing piece was designed describing the soon-to-be-printed products. This brochure was printed and mailed to approximately 17,000 addresses. It was also displayed along with all four publications at a meeting of the New York State Activities Association where sales were brisk. Note: An example of a judgement call which erred as too conservative was in the printing of the "Quizz-Whizz" packets.[4] Only 1000 were produced initially. Because of good sales, considerable money would have been saved if a larger quantity could have been printed initially. Estimating markets is still a difficult task. A valuable resource for the business of publishing is the Huenefeld Report.[5]

Expansion

In less than a year of operation the business was outgrowing its quarters. Luckily a nearby rental was found and business proceeded without much interruption.

At about the same time a decision was made to incorporate. The two main advantages were seen as (1) any liabilities incurred by a corporation cannot be claimed from the officers' personal income or possessions, (2) as a subchapter S corporation of the Internal Revenue Service Code, Section 1372, the firm's losses could be deducted from personal income to the extent of the shareholders' investment in the firm. The company was therefore incorporated under the laws of the State of New York and now became known as Potentials Development for Health and Aging Services, Inc.

More product material was constantly needed. Thus a number of steps were taken to supply it.

1. A listing in Writer's Market[6] was arranged.
2. Activity directors were contacted for ideas.
3. Authors of articles on related subjects in magazines were asked to expand these into books and booklets.
4. Therapists who presented relevant material at conferences were asked to develop their material for publication.
5. The elderly themselves wrote accounts about how they had met personal challenges.
6. A bibliography for activity directors was compiled.
7. More training and in-service education materials were developed.

The advantages of professional networking were illustrated by the result of a contact with a publisher of *Activities for the Frail Aged* in Edinburgh, Scotland. This book, useful to therapists, had been reviewed in the *American Journal of Occupational Therapy*. The author, now living in Australia, agreed to a U.S. edition of her book and that led to the distribution of Potentials Development materials in Australia. Subsequently orders from Ireland, the United Kingdom, Hong Kong, South Africa and Israel arrived showing the operation was now suddenly world-wide, a situation hardly dreamed of only two years previously.

By 1981 a book by another publisher was successfully added to the company's list and now (Summer 1984) eleven books by other publishers are distributed. The total number of publications listed has grown from the original four to fifty-nine. In addition, two films are available for rental. This rapidly increasing growth led to the constant need for more personnel, but by 1982 this need was stabilized and personnel were actually reduced by acquiring computerized services for mailing and invoicing and a payroll service to handle two salaried and four hourly employees in a cost-effective manner. In accordance with the owners' philosophy, paid staff range in age from 50 to 76 and all are women.

NEW VENTURES

Workshops

In March 1980 a new venture was added with the organization of an international conference on aging at which two dynamic Canadians were speakers along with U.S. presenters. Because of the enthusiastic acceptance of this conference, and an earlier session in 1979 in a children-of-aging-parents series, also successful, the owners decided to expand their activities to develop further educational offerings in which they would pursue three themes: "you and your aging parents," "sensitizing to the aged," and "creative aging."

Following a strategy used in the 1979 session, the second workshop model was developed employing as teaching techniques a delay feedback tape-recorder, a pair of oscillating goggles and a dozen pairs of cataract glasses, all used so that participants could actually experience the problems some older people have in communicating, relating to others and moving about. The model was initially used as a presentation at the Conference on Aging sponsored by the Buffalo Psychiatric Center. The method proved to be so beneficial and successful for learning that the material was transposed into a videotape, *Now That My World Is Small,*[7] through the production resources of the State University College at Buffalo. It subsequently had national exposure at the Annual Meeting of the Gerontological Society of America in 1982, and later at other national and regional meetings.

The third workshop model, on creative aging, resulted from demand in the fall of 1983 after a request from a church for an adult education series on aging. The sessions developed were well received, so now further development and implementation of this kind of workshop is in progress.

Slide/Tape Presentations

One success led to another when one of the authors had an experience with an elderly relative which tested her value judgements and raised questions about the rights of the elderly to control their own lives. A ninety year old aunt with failing judgement and memory wanted to marry another resident in her nursing home. He was considered "mentally incompetent." The author concluded that she was not the only one to face such situations and that there was doubtless a need for some educational/discussion vehicle to assist persons in thinking in a creative way about their own and their relatives' aging. The result was a slide/tape production designed to stimulate thinking by presenting situations which arise that test family and personal values. This too has been well received.

In-Service Education Services

Following the need which actually gave initial impetus to the business, the need for better training of persons working with the elderly, a number of materials and services have been created and are provided regularly. An in-service education series, called *People to People,* developed by a team including a registered nurse with an additional degree in rehabilitation counseling, a teacher and a registered occupational therapist, consists of 8 forty-five minute sessions and is given, when used in a facility, to staff of all three shifts by Potentials Development staff.

APPLYING A PHILOSOPHY IN A BUSINESS

From the start of the business the owners have believed in the objective of involving as many elders as possible as workers and volunteers in the operation. Initially at the "family and friend" stage, a ninety year old lady with an eighty-seven year old male friend came regularly for some months to the company offices to collate and package materials. Later, work was distributed to nursing home residents for which the home received a donation to its Activity Fund in return for the residents' help. Those who had collated and packaged materials collectively decided how the donated funds were to be spent. Such things as all going to a restaurant for a meal or all being able to take a bus trip have been made possible by this means. In addition, a general camaraderie not usually seen among residents in homes has resulted.

Some persons living in apartments for the elderly also enjoy this work for the same reasons. Other elderly persons have been sought to assist with speaking engagements, to relate various aspects of their personal aging experiences. For example, at a Senior Citizen Breakfast Club, sponsored by a local fast food restaurant with the program directed by Potentials Development staff, a couple in their late eighties and nineties, living in a nursing home, were encouraged to attend a series of these breakfasts. There they served as excellent role models and leaders since other participants were amazed to see these two persons at eight in the morning, attractively dressed, eager to participate, walking around, greeting others.

Further in the Breakfast Club project, the authors asked a lady in her eighties, who sews beautifully, to put together an advertising banner for the company to use. She also sewed table drapes and made the bag for ticket stubs for the drawing at each meeting when one person wins a copy of a book donated by the company. (This became a nice marketing strategy as well.)

In another aspect of the business, residents of a domiciliary facility helped make and decorate display boards for the company's materials and books that are shown at various events. Since these persons and many like them serve as adjunctive staff in the business, a picture album featuring all the elderly persons who sew, collate, and are part of workshops, in-service sessions and health fairs has been assembled. It now forms a regular part of the company's displays at meetings.

OTHER ACTIVITIES OF THE COMPANY

The owners decided to engage in various other community activities to benefit both elders and the continued growth of their business. In this mode, in the past two years a series of articles has been prepared for the *Golden Times,* a senior citizen newspaper of the Niagara Frontier. Titled *The Soul's Food,* the column features the lives of older persons who are continuing to serve others. Featured have been the lady who stitched the advertising banner, the participants in a creative writing class taught by one of the staff and a lady who crochets pins with seasonal themes and gives them to residents in long term care facilities.

The intent is to help readers to walk with pride through each day of the years ahead, enlarging their worlds by reaching out to others from wherever they are, confident that what they have to offer is acceptable and needed.

Through a *Sensitivity to Aging Workshop* that one of the authors led, an intergenerational project began—still one more facet of the business. Held in a church which has a large youth group, one of the youth group advisors who attended the workshop asked for a similar session for his young people to prepare them for what they would experience when they visited nursing homes to sing carols.

This led to teaching grammar school children about aging and to the development of one or two intergenerational projects for seventh and eighth grade students. Interesting results followed in which students made things the elders needed, and elders came to the school to express thanks. This encouraged continued visiting programs.

A second example of intergenerational strategies is a spring songfest held at a local school for which a seventh grader wrote words for a song about old and young persons needing each other. After her music teacher set the words to music, the song was included in the songfest. At the same time, the authors asked some seniors to write words for a "seniors song." A chorus of seniors from several senior centers were invited to sing their song at the same songfest. This resulted in many nice interchanges. This mutual participation was a big success, the songs were recorded on audio/video tape for the school and there was media coverage, including a photograph of the combined group in the local newspaper.

These kinds of successes involving children in learning about and working with older people led to the development of a curriculum unit for elementary schools to sensitize youngsters to the processes of aging. Because of part-time volunteer work on the project by a 4th grade teacher, and her enthusiasm for it, the resulting unit was accepted for field trial in her district. It was well received and is currently being edited for publication.

CONCLUSIONS

It is difficult to pinpoint results of all these ventures. Certainly there has been increased recognition in the Buffalo area for the needs of the elderly. Through participation and exposure to materials and staff nationally, the company's materials are now widely used by physicians, nurses, activity directors, occupational therapists and by the elderly themselves.

Certainly the scope of Potentials Development's activities has far exceeded early expectations of the owners. For example, the outreach to children of aging parents has produced a number of unexpected publications. Audiovisual materials have been produced and are in demand by colleges, junior colleges and nursing homes. Intergenerational developments show promise of expansion. However, a continued need for more capital to expand operations has been and remains a difficulty.

SUMMARY

The fact remains that two occupational therapists saw a need to effect change in attitudes about aging. Their work as consultants in nursing homes led to the formation of a company to produce practical educational materials. Start-up capital was available from the author. Later an elderly relative, together with others who shared the ideals of the therapists were willing to invest in the company. In six years the company had grown to a publishing business that sells materials by mail order all over the English speaking world. It has expanded to serve multi-generations through outreach and workshops as well as by published and audiovisual materials. While this discussion could not relate all the business aspects of the operation, it is hoped the descriptions of strategies of development and marketing will be helpful to others who are willing to risk, as the authors were, in pursuing a philosophy.

REFERENCES

1. DOK Publishers, Inc. 6 Russell Avenue, Buffalo, NY 14214
2. Deichman ES, Kirchhofer MV: *Working with the Elderly*, 1985 revision. Buffalo: Potentials Development
3. Out of print
4. Bohmer E: *Quizz Whizz*. Buffalo: Potentials Development
5. *The Huenefeld Report* Bedford, MA: The Huenefeld Co, Inc., PO Box U, 01730
6. *Writer's Market* Cincinnati, OH: Writer's Digest Books
7. *Now That My World Is Small* (3/4 A-V Cassette/27 min). Order from Film Librarian, Instructional Resources Center, State University College at Buffalo, 1300 Elmwood Ave., Buffalo, NY 14222

For further information on Potentials Development and the educational materials it produces, please contact Elizabeth S. Deichman at the company's office listed earlier in this paper.

Marketing
Occupational Therapy Services

Lisette N. Kautzmann, MS, OTR

ABSTRACT. The ability to understand and appropriately apply business skills is a key component in the development of a successful private practice. Marketing is one of the business skills occupational therapists need to have in order to take full advantage of the opportunities available to entrepreneurs in the health care industry. The purpose of this article is to present a structured approach to marketing occupational therapy services through the use of a marketing plan.

The four components of a marketing plan, a situation analysis, the identification of problems, opportunities, and target markets, the development of a marketing strategy for each targeted market, and a method to monitor the plan, are discussed. Applications to occupational therapy practice are suggested. The use of a marketing plan as a method for organizing and focusing marketing efforts is an effective means of supporting and enhancing the development of a private practice.

Recent changes in the health care system have provided opportunities and challenges for occupational therapists entering private practice. To successfully compete in this arena occupational therapists will need to integrate knowledge of sound business practices and clinical expertise. Marketing is one of the three business skills identified by Baum as critical for occupational therapy managers.[1] Effective marketing of occupational therapy services can influence the growth of the profession, communicate the importance of occupational therapy to targeted publics, and expand occupational therapy service delivery.[2] The purpose of this article is to present a struc-

Lisette N. Kautzmann is a doctoral candidate in Adult Education, Nova University.

This article appears jointly in *Private Practice in Occupational Therapy* (The Haworth Press, Inc., 1985), and *Occupational Therapy in Health Care*, Volume 2, Number 2 (Summer 1985).

91

tured approach to marketing occupational therapy services through the use of a marketing plan.

Marketing is defined as a human activity that is directed at satisfying needs and wants through an exchange process.[3] Typically this process involves the exchange of goods or services for a fair monetary gain. All organizations depend upon exchange relations to attract needed resources, convert them into useful products and services, and distribute them efficiently to target markets.[4] Marketing professionals agree that the exchange process should be directed and structured through the use of a marketing plan, which serves as the framework for all marketing efforts (see Table 1). There are four major components of a marketing plan: a situation analysis, identification of problems, opportunities, and target markets using information derived from the situation analysis, development of a marketing strategy for each target market, and a method to monitor the plan.

SITUATION ANALYSIS

The situation analysis is an examination of the external environment and the uncontrollable marketing variables. It is the basis for defining the private practice. The first step in a situation analysis is determination of the nature and extent of the demand for occupational therapy services. In assessing the demand or market it is important to identify all of the actual and potential buyers of occupational therapy services. Hospitals, schools, nursing homes, public health agencies, educational institutions, insurance carriers, and individuals are examples of buyers. Sources of data on actual and potential buyers of occupational therapy services include health systems agencies, public health agencies, and listings in the telephone directory yellow pages. This information establishes the broad perimeters of what might be possible in terms of a private practice. Awareness of the broad scope of the market provides a perspective for predicting trends and future needs in health care. The ability to perceive and act on these trends is vital to the success of a private practice.[5]

After the broad perimeters of practice are identified, the next step is to divide this market into homogeneous groups

Table 1

Components of a Marketing Plan

I. Situation analysis

    A. Nature and extent of demand

    B. Competition

    C. Environmental climate

    D. Clinical and management skills

    E. Financial resources

II. Problems and Opportunities

    A. Identification of target market segments

III. Marketing strategy

    A. Objectives

        1. Volume

        2. Profit

    B. Marketing mix implementation strategies

        1. Product strategy

        2. Place strategy

        3. Price strategy

        4. Promotion strategy

            a. Personal selling

            b. Mass selling

                1). Advertising

                2). Publicity

            c. Sales promotion

IV. Monitoring

    A. Attainment of objectives

    B Effectiveness of marketing mix

through market segmentation. Marketing professionals use geographic, demographic, psychographic, and behavioral variables to segment a market. Geographic variables describe community characteristics. Demographic variables relate to the personal characteristics of the consumer such as age, sex, family size, income level, occupation, religion, and nationality. Psychographic variables are the consumer's social class and life style. Behavioral variables include consumer knowledge, use, attitude, and response to a product.[3] These and other variables are useful to occupational therapists. Geographic variables identify the geographic and physical location of service delivery. Opportunities and challenges in rural settings differ from those in urban communities and service delivery in acute care hospitals differs from school system practice. Reimbursement variables refer to the purchase of health care and include Medicare, Medicaid, private insurance, worker's compensation, and self-pay. Two of the most important variables for occupational therapists are the demographic variables of client age and diagnosis. Therapists frequently view their practice as a reflection of their clinical skills and identify themselves as hand therapists or school therapists. This can be an effective way to segment the market, particularly when it is combined with the geographic and reimbursement variables.

Once the market segments have been established each segment should be analyzed in terms of the current level of service and competition. The Administration Special Interest Sections of state occupational therapy associations, state occupational therapy association offices, and networking with other therapists and health professionals are sources of information on level of service and competition. This analysis will identify gaps in service delivery and underserved populations in each market segment. It also will serve as an information source on who is providing services to each market segment and possible reasons for the lack of service delivery.

The next step in the situation analysis is an environmental scan of the external factors affecting each market segment. Marketing professionals include political and legal, social and cultural, competitive, economic and technological factors, and resources.[6] Occupational therapists are particularly influenced by factors relating to reimbursement. Practice has changed dramatically in institutions that are paid prospectively for service. This has a significant impact on private practitioners who are considering providing contractual service to these institutions. In these settings occupational therapy is viewed as a cost. Thus, occupational therapists must demonstrate that they contribute to improvement in function, decreased length of stay, and movement of patients through a vertical system of health care. Legal constraints, regulations, and professional guidelines define the type and level of occupational therapy service delivery in a variety of settings such as home health agencies, nursing homes, schools, and programs for chronic mentally ill. Examples of these constraints and regulations include federal Medicare regulations, state licensure and Medicaid requirements, and American Occupational Therapy Association (AOTA) Standards of Practice and Principles of Occupational Therapy Ethics.

The final component of the situation analysis is an assessment of personal skills and financial resources. Matching the clinical and management competencies required for each of the market segments with personal abilities results in information on one's strengths and weaknesses and identifies additional training and credentialing needs. Although a full discussion of financial planning is beyond the scope of this article, the financial requirements of each market segment should be estimated. Considerations such as the need to equip a clinic, rent an office, hire assistants and clerical help, and use of a personal car for home visits must be identified and weighed against the potential for reimbursement. Further information on financial planning is included in the AOTA *Private Practice Information Packet*[5] and the May 1984 issue of the *American Journal of Occupational Therapy*.

PROBLEMS AND OPPORTUNITIES

The situation analysis provides an in-depth view of the business and practice requirements for each market segment. Factors identified included the demand for service, competition, external factors affecting practice, personal and financial resources and information regarding clientele to be served, the income potential, the amount of time required to generate the desired amount of revenue, and the potential for growth in each market segment. This information is used to examine the problems and opportunities associated with each market segment. It is the foundation of the decision making process regarding selection of target market and when and where to enter the market.

The process of identifying the most favorable or advantageous segments of a specific market and directing efforts to meet their needs by developing a marketing mix strategy for each identified segment is called target marketing.[6] Target marketing is advantageous because it places sellers in a position to spot market opportunities and fine tune their product, pricing, and promotional efforts to match the needs of the targeted market.[3]

MARKETING STRATEGY

Marketing strategy includes objectives and implementation strategies for each targeted market. Specific profit and volume objectives with time frames for achievement are operationalized through the development of a marketing mix strategy for each target market. This approach allows the private practitioner to custom design his or her marketing efforts and practice to meet the needs and desires of targeted clientele. The marketing mix has four components: product, place, price, and promotion.[6] These are controllable marketing variables and are considered equally important to the success of a target marketing effort.

The product component of the marketing mix is a combination of goods and services that meets the needs of the targeted buyers.[6] Goods and services can include physical objects, services, persons, places, organizations, and ideas.[3] The occupational therapy product is the skills of the individual therapist in the roles of clinician, manager, consultant, educator, and researcher. Central to the exchange process and the success of the marketing effort is the quality of the product and its attunement to the needs and desires of the targeted public. Special training, education, experience, and credentialing in the skills and services required by the targeted publics are vital for product credibility. This training and experience then becomes a selling point in the promotional aspect of the marketing mix. Quality assurance and efficacy studies further substantiate the effectiveness and value of occupational therapy services.

The manner in which the product is distributed is the "place" component of the marketing mix.[6] For occupational therapists in private practice, place is where occupational therapy services are provided. In addition to the traditional institution and school locations patients also may be treated in the community. An office that is maintained by a therapist independently or shared with physicians or other health professionals, private homes, wellness centers, and medical-surgical centers that are being built in or near shopping malls are community sites for the delivery of occupational therapy services.

Occupational therapy services must be easily accessible to the targeted clientele. Transportation to the location should be readily available. If the consumers routinely receive multidisciplinary treatment, then the place where occupational therapy services are delivered should be in the proximity of other service providers. Availability of parking is a consideration when outpatients are treated. Well-run, uncrowded, professional appearing physical facilities create an atmosphere that is conducive to customer satisfaction. Customer satisfaction is a major marketing goal because it indicates that the targeted consumer is convinced of the value of the exchange process and can give positive feedback on services received to referral sources and potential consumers.

Price is the exchange value of goods and services.[3] In the health care industry this usually is a monetary exchange. Consumers and third party payers are increasingly aware of the differences in the cost of services. Thus, private practitioners must be able to meet competitors' prices. Many state association Administration Special Interest Sections have compiled information on usual charges for service. Frequently, rates of reimbursement for occupational therapists, physical therapists, and speech pathologists are similar in Medicare and Medicaid programs and may be used as comparison sources. Methods for setting fees are described in the AOTA *Private Practice Information Packet,*[5] the *Product Output Reporting System and Uniform Terminology,*[7] and by Hershman in her article on private practice reimbursement.[8]

Promotion is the communication of information between the seller and the buyer.[3] It is how you tell your targeted market about your product, place, and price. Personal selling, mass selling, and sales promotion are the three components of promotion.

Personal selling is face-to-face communication between the seller and the buyer.[6] It is the most expensive yet most effective form of promotion. Occupational therapists use personal selling as their primary promotional method. It is the one tool that all thearpists will need to use in building a private practice. There are two groups to whom private practitioners must convey the value of occupational therapy services: the referral sources and the consumers or consumer representatives. Since the services offered must compliment and augment the needs and desires of the referral source or consumer, the personal selling presentation of the product, place, and price should be specifically designed to meet the needs and desires of the target market. In planning the presentation decide what information is to be conveyed and what is to be achieved. Practice delivering that information in a clear, concise manner. Support the presentation with promotional literature such as the AOTA Professional Profile, annual calendar, efficacy studies or personal promotional brochure to emphasize the value of occupational therapy services. Afterwards assess whether or not the goals of the presentation were met, how it might be improved, and what type of follow-up is indicated.

Examples of other types of personal selling include: serving as either a paid or unpaid lecturer or "guest expert" in health care education, participating in health fairs, serving on boards or committees of public health agencies, conducting health screenings, and participating in continuing education and in-service presentations with other health professionals. AOTA has developed several public information video tapes and films that can be used to enhance these presentations.

Mass selling is communicating with large numbers of consumers at the same time and includes advertising and publicity.[6] Advertising is any paid form of nonpersonal presentation of ideas, goods, or services by an identified sponsor.[3] Publicity is free editorial space or time.[3] Examples of mass selling are magazines ads, television commercials, posters, brochures, and catalogues. Information on how to use mass selling techniques is included in the AOTA publication *Public Relations on Target for OT.*[9]

Direct mail to targeted buyers is a highly effective form of advertising.[10] Development of a direct mail brochure describing the services offered to each targeted market and a summary of therapist qualifications, address, and telephone number is recommended. Private practitioners also should list themselves in the telephone directory yellow and white pages. AOTA guidelines for advertising are presented in the Principles of Occupational Therapy Ethics.[11]

> Advertising by therapists under their professional title shall be in accordance with propriety and precedent in health professions.
>
> *Guidelines:* Occupational therapists may provide information to the public about available services through procedures established by the employing facility or contracting agency. If an occupational therapist provides an independent service, it is appropriate to advertise those services.
>
> The occupational therapist shall not use, or participate in the use of, any form of communication containing a false, fraudulent, misleading, deceptive, self-laudatory or unfair statement or claim. Testimonials or statements which promise a favorable result shall be avoided.

Publicity is another mass selling means of gaining public attention. Activities that are open to the public and in the public interest attract publicity. Thus, participation in prevention, wellness, and educational activities can result in heightened public awareness of the services provided by a private practitioner. Therapists may have to write their own press releases and submit them to the news media. The positive aspect of publicity is that it is free; however, the individual therapist has little control over it and it often is difficult to focus publicity on specific target markets.

Sales promotion is the use of short term incentives to encourage purchase or sale of a product or service.[3] Consumer promotion incentives include coupons, discounts, samples, premiums, and contests. Sales promotion incentives are beginning to emerge as marketing tools in the health care industry. They are used primarily by institutions such as hospitals and medical-surgical centers. Examples of these incentives are discounts for using hospital facilities during slack times, newspaper coupons for free blood pressure and diabetes screening, and free informational lecture and phone messages on health and disease topics. Occupational therapists will need to develop an awareness of trends in the use of incentives and examine their compliance with ethical practice.

MONITORING THE PLAN

Monitoring is the systematic use of checks to ascertain progress toward the achievement of objectives and the introduction of corrective action when necessary.[4] In addition, periodic examination of the effectiveness of each of the marketing mix elements, in relation to the targeted markets, is advisable. Private practitioners can send out follow-up letters and questionnaires to referral sources and consumers asking for feedback on the marketing mix and specific promotional efforts. Close attention to attainment or lack of attainment of the predetermined volume and profit objectives and time lines is vital to the health of the private practice.

SUMMARY

The use of an organized plan to structure the marketing efforts of the private practitioner was presented. A situation analysis was used to examine the external marketing variables and approaches to segmenting the market. This was followed by application of the information derived from the situation analysis to identification of problems, opportunities, and target markets. Marketing strategies, including objectives and the marketing mix for target markets, were described and applications to occupational therapy practice were suggested. Careful monitoring of progress in attaining the marketing objectives and the effectiveness of the marketing mix strategies was emphasized. The marketing plan represents a solid framework for occupational therapists to use in organizing and focusing their marketing efforts in a manner that supports and enhances the development of a private practice.

REFERENCES

1. Baum CM: Power, Politics, Persuasion: Growth Strategies for the 80's. An institute presented at the 64th annual American Occupational Therapy Association Conference, Kansas City, 1984.

2. Baum CM: Strategic Integrated Management System-SIMS. Am J Occup Ther 37: 595–600, 1983.

3. Kotler P: Principles of Marketing. Englewood Cliffs, NJ: Prentice-Hall, 1980

4. Kotler P: Marketing for Nonprofit Organizations. Englewood Cliffs, NJ: Prentice-Hall, 1975.

5. Division of Practice: Private Practice Information Packet. Rockville, MD: American Occupational Therapy Association, 1982.

6. McCarthy JE: Basic Marketing, 7th Edition. Homewood, IL: Richard D. Irwin, 1981.

7. Commission on Practice: Occupational Therapy Product Output Reporting System and Uniform Terminology for Reporting Occupational Therapy Services. Rockville, MD: American Occupational Therapy Association, 1979.

8. Hershman AG: Reimbursement in Private Practice. Am J Occup Ther 38: 299–306, 1984.

9. ————: Public Relations on Target for OT. Rockville, MD: American Occupational Therapy Association, 1976.

10. Olson TS: Power, Politics, Persuasion: Growth Strategies for the 80's An institute presented at the 64th annual American Occupational Therapy Association Conference, Kansas City, 1984.

11. Commission on Standards and Ethics: Principles of Occupational Therapy Ethics. Rockville, MD: American Occupational Therapy Association, 1980.

Computers and the Private Practitioner in Occupational Therapy

Estelle Breines, MA, OTR, FAOTA

ABSTRACT. Computer application to the area of occupational therapy practice is a relatively recent undertaking. Because of the absence of pertinent literature, suggestions given for potential uses are derived from imagination and from recent experience. As a therapist in private practice, concerned with cost and efficiency as well as quality treatment, the computer is examined as an administrative and research tool. Therapists are given guidelines so as to choose whether and where to initiate computer use. Next, computers and tasks are subjected to activity analysis, suggesting adaptations for use and proposing some treatment applications. Potential hazards and future needs are discussed, including computer literacy in education of therapists, compatibility of hardware/software, and communication between therapists.

If one had been born at home; walked great distances to school; travelled by horse drawn vehicles; learned a trade from one's parents; lived through several wars to end all wars, with ever increasing technology for both health and destruction; saw the birth of cars, planes, rockets and satellites; experienced stereopticons, silent films, talkies, and video cassettes; saw the communications media develop from newspapers to television, one supposes then, that the magic of computers would not be any more difficult to conceive than

Estelle Breines is President of Geri-Rehab, Inc., of Lebanon, N.J. She is a Doctoral Student and Teaching Fellow in the Occupational Therapy Department at New York University.

Acknowledgement: This paper was prepared and edited on a TRS-80 II using SCRIPSIT software.

This article appears jointly in *Private Practice in Occupational Therapy* (The Haworth Press, Inc., 1985), and *Occupational Therapy in Health Care,* Volume 2, Number 2 (Summer 1985).

were all those happenings. Computers are one more new experience.

Today computers impact upon us all. They are used in business, in supermarkets, in design and engineering. One cannot envision the scope of computer use in the future, in general, or as applied to health care. Computer application is bounded only by imagination and creativity.

Since creativity is the stock in trade of occupational therapy, it is only appropriate that occupational therapists should begin to address the application of computers to the settings in which they operate and to the care of the populations they serve. One such setting is a private practice business, Geri-Rehab, Inc. In this paper, the writer will describe the experience of her company in using a Radio Shack TRS-80 Model II Micro Computer (Model II) for both administrative and treatment purposes. By so doing, it is hoped other therapists with relatively small-scale operations will see potentials in the use of computers for their setting or population.

ADMINISTRATIVE TOOL

In order to meet the needs of cost effectiveness, to heighten efficiency, maximize time utilization and aid in research, Geri-Rehab, Inc. investigated the computer market and selected Model II. This selection was based upon several concerns. This equipment enabled the use of a variety of readily available software. Service and supplies are also readily available, since Radio Shack stores are located within close proximity to our rurally situated office, and many others are not. This choice has never been regretted.

Using a Model II with one expansion disk drive, a Daisy Wheel Printer II and *SCRIPSIT* (Tandy, 1981), the Radio Shack version of word processing, Geri-Rehab, Inc. has been able to correspond, bill patients, retain and retrieve consultation reports, develop grant proposals, maintain and update procedures manuals, keep contracts current, and typeset publications and promotional material. Word processing software allows keyed instructions to be sent to the computer to tell the printer to provide "hard" or paper copies of selected information. Printing output can be varied in infinite ways by altering the parameters of instructions and by the many printing options available. For example, reports, labels, lists, type setting and other applications are possible with appropriate formatting.

PAYROLL (Tandy, 1982) permits checks to be drawn with automatic computations for withholding, and prepares weekly, monthly and year end statements and W2 forms. *VISICALC*, (Radio Shack, 1980) an accounting spread sheet, is used to prepare facilities' bills, itemizing and computing individual patient treatment charges for each facility with which Geri-Rehab, Inc. contracts. Lists have been prepared with the use of *PROFILE* II (Tandy, 1981), which permits sorting by zip code, alphabet, and special categories, enabling the production of mailing labels and reports. This has been a considerable assist in the distribution of our publications.

Using the *DATASTAR* (MicroPro, 1983) and *REPORT-STAR* (Micropro, 1983) data base management system programs together with the *PICKLES and TROUT* (1983) version of the CP/M operating system, software has been developed to collect data about patient performance generated by the *Functional Assessment Scale* (Breines, 1983). When complete, this package will permit sorting by any number of categories. It has been programmed for use with the *Functional Assessment Scale* to sort by diagnosis, facility, therapist, and guarantor, enabling the results to be further analyzed by statistical software. Preliminary statistical analysis indicated that age of elderly subjects studied was not a factor in performance competency, so age was not chosen as a sorting criteria, thus providing more disk space and efficiency for data storage of significant items. Careful analysis of real information needs contributes to economical utilization of data, equipment and time—all of which represent cost.

Geri-Rehab, Inc., has recently acquired a modem. This will enable us to link by telephone with other data banks for both information and research. Until the equipment is fully on line, one cannot imagine all the ways it will be of use. Our most recent acquisition is the TRS-80 Model 100. This portable computer fits into a handbag the size of a small briefcase. It has full word processing capability. This computer is designed to hook up with the Model II. It has expanded our capabilities beyond our expectations. Operated by either battery or house current, it serves as a second keyboard when the Model II is in use. It is used for note taking at meetings, and stores schedules and phone numbers. It contains its own modem, so data can be transmitted to the Model II by phone from any point away from the office. This capability is ideal for a practice which is largely itinerant. On several occasions it has been used with patients in their own homes.

COMPUTER, AN ADMINISTRATIVE TOOL FOR YOU?

In determining the value of computer applications versus traditional applications, it is necessary for the potential user to weigh the investment of money and time. To familiarize oneself with a software package for administration takes many hours. If the usefulness of the package is limited, it may be better to retain traditional methods. If, on the other hand, the job which will be facilitated is expected to come up repeatedly, the speed and accuracy which the computer affords will certainly make the start-up costs well worth the time spent. The uses to which the computer is applied in the Geri-Rehab, Inc., office continue to expand daily. Expansion is limited only by the time available to develop new applications.

COMPUTER AS OCCUPATIONAL THERAPY TOOL

The computer is a tool of the present and the future. It has structured lives today to a greater extent than yet realized. Still, the computer remains a mystery, requiring imagination in conceptualizing its use in therapeutic practice. Little documentation on the application of computers to occupational therapy has as yet reached the professional literature. Because of this dearth of information, it would be interesting and valuable to reflect on the role the computer will take in the field. Therefore, much of what is to be addressed must be gleaned from the therapist's imagination and very current practice experience. The analysis is less than scientific, but will hopefully seed the creativity of others.

To use any tool for occupational therapy, it is first necessary to subject that tool and its associated activities to analysis. Restricting the attention of this paper to the personal or small business computer, the unit to be discussed is one which is self-contained, runs on ordinary household electrical current, has a viewing screen and a keyboard, and may or may not have peripheral equipment such as expansion disk drives, a printer or a modem. The viewing screen is similar to a television monitor, often referred to by users as a CRT or cathode ray tube. The CRT permits communications to be monitored visually. Screens on some equipment can be modified so that they print black on white or white on black. Some screens are green or amber, colors which some manufacturers claim is less apt to cause eye strain. Black and white screens can be adapted by placing a colored filter onto the glass of the CRT.

Those who are uninitiated may begin to understand computers by comparing them with other tools with which they are more familiar. Depending upon its application, the computer can be used as a superbly efficient typewriter, a sophisticated calculator, an art medium, a game board, an auxiliary memory, a compact filing cabinet, an educator and perhaps several other things which escape the understanding of this writer. And, remarkably, the same piece of equipment can do all these things with no more adaptation than one ordinarily applies when one changes a record on a record player.

The computer is a communication instrument ordinarily spoken to through a keyboard, but is subject to modification if necessary, such as by the use of puff-and-sip equipment or other such activator devices (Wamboldt, 1984). It is a tool which can be applied to the frivolous as well as to the complex, just as a typewriter can be used to write a letter to a friend or a significant document. In order to do either, one is not required to know much more about the instrument's use than how to start it up, put the paper in, and strike the keys. Of course, the more one knows about the tool and the principles of its design, the more flexibility and potential the instrument provides.

Because it lends itself to a variety of adaptations and applications, the computer makes an ideal tool for the occupational therapist. As a computer's keyboard is essentially designed like that of a typewriter, it is subject to those adaptations ordinarily used to adapt typewriters. Among these are head wands, keyboard guards, and the like. Unlike the typewriter, some computer equipment offers the advantage of alternative positioning of the keyboard apart from the main body of the equipment. The light-weight keyboard on much equipment is portable. When attached by a cable to the computer, the keyboard can be removed from a stationary site adjacent to the computer and placed in a position at which it may be more easily reached by individuals restricted in mobility or access. Mobility of equipment components provides much more flexibility in positioning than is ordinarily available even with a standard portable typewriter. Portability of the entire equipment between locations makes other adaptations possible. Communication can also occur between computers by using modems which use telephone hookups. Distance is virtually unlimited.

By making the computer a tool of practice, it can become a vehicle by which the occupational therapist can transit practice from the industrial to the technological/electronic era. For the therapist in private practice it becomes an essential tool for running an efficient and profitable business. The computer can be used in treatment for a variety of purposes. It is an excellent communication tool for the non-verbal patient who has retained other expressive language skills. In addition to screen displays, some sophisticated computers have vocal simulators which can be used with individuals who are unable to produce meaningful vocalizations.

The computer is ideal for the patient who finds non-dominant handwriting a chore or is discouraged by inadequate handwriting. Unlike the typewriter, errors are easily corrected. This feature of easy correction permits the patient to produce a clean and attractively printed product despite severe dysfunction.

Customarily, speed and accuracy increase rapidly once anxiety is eliminated. It is fun to see mistakes disappear with the strike of a key. This error elimination feature is valuable for patients with cognitive and perceptual disorders. Because of the ease with which errors can be corrected, the computer, configured for word processing, can be used effectively as a tool for teaching finger gnosia and fine motor skills. Word processing permits patients to send letters to families, enables copy to be retained by patients, and permits material to be read and corrected by therapists or by patients themselves at a later date. Patients can be provided with their own discs and can be encouraged to independently use the equipment for practice during periods when patients and equipment are free.

Because the computer is an exciting instrument which provides no limit to the mind expansion and skill building it permits, it is ideal for the cardiac or respiratory patient who is restricted in energy expenditure. It is a craft in every sense of the word. It delivers a creative product for which satisfaction is engendered, while creating an energy demand which is modest.

Coordination, speed, and accuracy are skills individuals develop through the use of computer games in the arcades with which we are all familiar. These goals are appropriate for many patients as well, and can be achieved through the use of game software.

Some game playing requires the use of a joystick. Our staff has successfully adapted an Atari joystick with K Splint in a modified C bar design to sustain the thumb in opposition for a hemiplegic patient. This permitted the patient to play computer games while reinforcing opposition. Use of the splint during play resulted in the gradual elimination of the adaptation and ultimate acquisition of competent three jaw chuck grasp and a fully functional hand.

These are only a few ideas of many that will assuredly be generated in time, as our experience with computers grows. Undoubtedly, in time, many other adaptations will derive from the problems which will present themselves to patients and therapists. Geri-Rehab, Inc., can only expect that as computer use increases, its use will reflect favorably upon our patients.

RESTRICTIONS ON USE

Some concerns about computer use generate from the fact that the computer is a very compelling instrument. Once engrossed in the problem solving it permits, time eludes one. Meals go uneaten, sleep is irregular, family is unheeded. While mind expanding, it is, however, a static, immobile activity and therefore potentially incapacitating for the elderly or others with limited endurance. Like the mother who dictates, "Enough TV. Go out and play", the same dictum holds here.

Following this line of thinking, it may be a risk to emphasize the use of computers in the resolution of perceptual and cognitive disorders. The computer screen is two-dimensional. Two-dimensional arrays are abstractions of three-dimensional experience and may be dependent upon depth for meaningful perception to be created. Bear in mind as well that sedentary tasks offer no stimulation to the periphery of the visual field. Only the foveal fields of vision are stimulated. Therefore, opportunities for the resolution of perception of spatial dimensions are restricted. Such perceptual resolutions are dependent upon the synthesis of stimulus data from peripheral and foveal visual fields in the dimensional world (Trevarthen, 1968; Breines, 1981). While computers are being used by cognitive training programs, because of the concerns cited above, the premises upon which these programs are provided warrant further theoretical analysis and demonstrated worth. The use of a two-dimensional tool for the resolution of a problem which derives from a three-dimensional dysfunction requiring peripheral input, may heighten rather than resolve perceptual disorders, or may resolve problems in a splinter skill fashion, rather than address underlying causes of the problem.

 Both lack of mobility and resultant sensory deprivation have been shown to result in disorientation even in normal young adults (Zuckerman, 1969). One might conclude that if normal, well, young people are potentially at risk, individuals with sensitive and fragile nervous systems may be subject to similar dysfunctions without caution exercised. That the elderly are subject to nervous system disorders is well documented. Therefore, they as well as younger disabled persons may be populations at risk of disorientation or other cognitive disorders through immobility associated with computer use. These issues will need to be monitored and assessed to determine their relevance, as our experience with computers grows. The need to assess this matter is suggested as a research topic.

Another concern may be the constant visual stimulation associated with computer use. Working people have been known to report that continual use of the computer as a job related tool causes eyestrain and headaches. One cannot anticipate the responses of a cataract prone or neurologically impaired population to computer use without further investigation.

Personal experience alerted the author to a potential problem for individuals who wear bifocal corrective lenses. In bifocals, the near vision corrective field is in the lower frame of the eyeglasses. The upper frame is corrected for distance vision. The individual wearing bifocals is subject to experiencing neck discomfort when he attempts to see more clearly by extending the neck to read the screen through the lower frame, or taking the other option, experiencing eyestrain by keeping the head neutrally positioned while viewing the screen through the improperly focused upper frame. Neither solution is comfortable or recommended. To remediate this problem, reading or near vision glasses were purchased for explicit use with the computer. The eyeglasses are stored in the drawer of the computer desk so they are always available. Since use of bifocals is common for the elderly, this is a concern to which the therapist must be alert when instructing the older patient in computer use.

EFFICACY EFFECTS

While isolation, lack of sensory stimulation and eye strain associated with computer use are potential hazards of which one must be aware, many potential benefits can also be engendered. One is the sense of accomplishment which derives from the acquisition of skills held in high repute. The value of the computer as a creative tool is inordinate. The feedback obtained from others, for accomplishments exhibited in computer use, results in improved self-image.

Another positive benefit is the sense of camaraderie of belonging to the computer-wise "in" folk, or even more directly, being able to converse through modems with other operators with similar interests, thus potentially expanding the vistas of a population which is often limited in its ability to get around in the community. Special interest computer clubs abound. These clubs can provide social opportunities where other social experiences are ordinarily infeasible.

PROGRAM WRITING

Nowhere in this paper has program writing been previously addressed. One is able to successfully own and use a computer without even being familiar with computer languages or how to write programs, although capabilities in this area would assuredly expand the usefulness of the equipment for individuals and for the profession as a whole. As yet, few occupational therapists have addressed themselves to software or program design, undoubtedly because few have the necessary programming skills to meet these needs. While programming is perhaps not a skill demanded of everyone, there is a real need for some occupational therapists to acquire competency in programming and computer languages, so that specialized requirements can be met by individuals who are computer experts and occupational therapists as well.

IMAGINED APPLICATIONS

Imagination enables conjecture about the uses one can conceive for the future. One can envision hooking up a wide television screen such as is available in some nursing homes, enabling groups to participate in some computer application, perhaps an interfacility computer olympics. Cooperation and competition could be devised in arcade style games, simulated bowling and football, error finding puzzles, creative writing, graphics and other such events. Another valuable use for the computer would be to establish a daily call system to at-risk elders in the community.

Due to increased longevity and anticipated long years of good health, the years of employment may be assumed to be increasing. People often retire to new vocations, rather than retire from old careers. Because flexible employment hours and computer skills are compatible, those trained in computer skills may find part-time employment opportunities in their own homes. Such employment may provide work opportunities which are compatible with reduced energy needs sometimes required by the disabled. The days of cottage industry may have returned.

These are only a few ideas of many that will assuredly be generated in time, as our experience with computers grows.

FUTURE CONSIDERATIONS

Several areas will have to be addressed by the occupational therapy profession in the near future if computer application is to continue to expand for practice. These are the development of more direct practice tools and the strategies for the accumulation of data from practice.

It remains for the therapists to design specialized programs to be used for resolving individual patient problems, such as tracking, word and letter recognition, sequencing, categorization, cognitive mapping, utilizing fine motor skills, ad infinitum. In addition, the problems of incompatibility of hardware and software among users needs resolution. Therapists all over the country have computers and software which cannot be shared. Software programs are designed by their manufacturers for use on specific equipment. For example, now* IBM and APPLE software cannot be interchanged. Therefore, therapists tend to function in isolation one from the other, as incompatibility of software between users has prevented sharing things they have developed. Therapists need to know who has compatible wares and to establish communication with them, so as to expand their vistas and improve treatment. The identification of and development of software "translators" will enhance communication, and speed the resolution of problems presently being addressed by individuals in isolation.

In terms of research, occupational therapists who work in private practice have the ideal tool with which to gather data to prove their cost effectiveness. Occupational therapists live in a commercial world in which data collection and economics are inextricably tied to governmental decisions regarding health care. Occupational therapists must begin to justify their practice, and with the aid of the computer, can do so. If the computer can be used to aid in validating occupational therapy, patients themselves stand to benefit from such research.

---

*At the time this article was prepared, November 1984.

Finally, in order to prepare future therapists with the skills they will need, occupational therapy educational programs must obtain and operate computers in their classes to familiarize students and faculty with applications in management, treatment, and research.

PROFESSIONAL COMMUNICATION

To their credit, occupational therapists have begun to recognize these problems and needs. Attempts to communicate their interests and capabilities have begun to be demonstrated. The organizational meeting of the Occupational Therapy Computer Club held in Portland, Oregon in May of 1983 indicated a recognition on the part of some therapists that more in the profession must be aware, exchange ideas, and develop applications. The 1984 AOTA Conference in Kansas City demonstrated an active response to the considerable number of computer programs available. Therapists were overheard to speak knowledgeably about bits and bytes and discs and drives, about courses in BASIC, FORTRAN, and COBOL, about computer activated adaptive equipment, and about research data collection. Therapists are studying and practicing their new craft, developing data collection systems, and sharing solutions. They are breaking new ground by addressing their expertise to the needs of their clients and colleagues.

SUMMARY

The use of computers by therapists in private practice can be a most positive and efficient addition to the daily routine and to the successful expansion of both business and treatment aspects of an operation. The profession must continue to expand its expertise so as to advance computer applicability in occupational therapy through the exchange of information, and education of new and experienced therapists.

Occupational therapists are entering a new technological era. As the era unfolds, the computer will be a health care tool, just as it is becoming a tool in other industries. It behooves the occupational therapist to learn to use this tool skillfully in the same way that they have learned to use other tools of practice.

REFERENCES

1. ————. *SCRIPSIT* 2.0 Program (1981) Ft. Worth: Tandy Corp.

2. ————. *PAYROLL* (1982) Ft. Worth: Tandy Corp.

3. Software Arts, Inc. *VISICALC* (1980) Ft. Worth: Radio Shack, Tandy Corp.

4. ————. *PROFILE II PROGRAM* (1981) Ft. Worth: Tandy Corp.

5. ————. *DataStar Release 1.4* (1982) San Raphael, CA: MicroPro International

6. ————. *ReportStar 1.0* (1982) San Raphael, CA: MicroPro International

7. ————. *P & T CP/M 2 Version 2.2m floppy* (1983) Goleta, CA: Pickles & Trout

8. Breines, E (1983) *Functional Assessment Scale* Lebanon, NJ: Geri-Rehab

9. Wamboldt, J Computer applications in treatment *OTHC* #1–4 Nov. 1984

10. Trevarthen, C (1968) Vision in fish: The origins of the visual frame for action in vertebrates. In Ingle, D (Ed.) *The Central Nervous System* Chicago: U. of Chicago Press

11. Breines, E (1981) *Perception: Its Development and Recapitulation* Lebanon, NJ: Geri-Rehab

12. Zuckerman, M (1969) Hallucinations: Reported sensations and image, in Zubek, J (Ed.) *Sensory Deprivation: Fifteen Years of Research* NY: Appleton-Century Crofts

Wellness:
Its Myths, Realities,
and Potential
for Occupational Therapy

Jerry A. Johnson, EdD, OTR, FAOTA

ABSTRACT. The paper presents some of the accepted interpretations of wellness and defines "context" preparatory to an
exploration of wellness. Secondly, it discusses a cultural shift
in our society that brings forth the possibility of wellness as a
context for living. Finally, it provides some thoughts about the
potential for occupational therapy in the area of wellness and
its implications for our practice.

Interpretations of wellness abound. Insurance companies
generally view wellness as a responsibility to be assumed by
individuals that will reduce the insurance company's medical
payments. However, the majority of insurance companies do
not pay for wellness programs because they are considered to
be either educational or "unscientific"—unsupported by research. Furthermore, payment for wellness programs is limited in that it has been difficult to prove that an illness or
disease has been prevented.

The paper is adapted from a presentation made at the Fall Symposium of the
Center for the Study of Sensory Integrative Dysfunction, September 24–25, Los
Angeles, California.

Dr. Jerry A. Johnson is founder and President of Context, Incorporated (a resource center for health and well-being), Denver, Colorado. She is nationally known
as an occupational therapy leader, educator, researcher and innovator. The Center,
and its programs, embodies some of her convictions about the future of occupational
therapy.

The author wishes to acknowledge the contributions made by Harriet M. Schmid,
PhD, OTR, in the preparation of this paper. Her thoughts and support are greatly
appreciated.

This article appears jointly in *Private Practice in Occupational Therapy* (The
Haworth Press, Inc., 1985), and *Occupational Therapy in Health Care*, Volume 2,
Number 2 (Summer 1985).

Hospitals with "wellness" programs frequently offer a variety of health promotion programs directed at weight loss, smoking cessation, exercise, nutrition, and/or stress. While these programs are not consistent with each other in philosophy or approach, many are based on the perspective of pathology, disease, and symptom management, with a focus on content rather than context.

The medical community is generally skeptical about "wellness" in that most studies of associations between lifestyle and diagnosis have been established only after a disease process is well established.

Contributing to the confusion surrounding the term wellness are the many individuals who offer "wellness" programs. Many of these individuals include persons who have had life-altering experiences and who want to share that experience with others. Other providers of "wellness" include retailers of vitamins and food supplements, and some are operators of exercise or weight loss clinics. Some health professionals are using a variety of unscientific techniques (e.g., techniques which have little support from research studies). Other health professionals clearly believe that wellness, or health, is a function of integration of mind, body, and spirit.

Business applies the terms wellness to health promotion programs that contribute to improved health, reduced absenteeism and medical claims, and improved productivity by employees. In fact, the greatest clarity about the wellness concept is found in the business community, whose objectives for wellness and health promotion programs include:

1. Increased productivity: that is, better quality of work, more units of work produced, higher morale, reduced absenteeism, and perhaps lower health care costs;
2. Cost savings: less sick time, and reductions in payment for employee health insurance claims; and
3. Improved Public Relations: such as better corporate image, favorable media coverage for employee health promotion programs, and statements by prospective employees that the company's health promotion programs were among their incentives for wanting to affiliate with the company.[1]

The President of the Health Insurance Association of America said: "Suffice it to say that wellness programs at the worksite are no passing fad. They are an integral part of management strategy to improve productivity and, over time, trim the costs of doing business."[2]

A point to note is that not once is improvement in employee health listed as an objective.

WELLNESS DEFINED

What then is wellness? A search of three dictionaries yielded no definitions. Review of many articles produced descriptions of programs, but again no definitions. Finally, in reviewing *Time Magazine's* Special Advertising Section on June 18, 1984, I found the following:

Wellness could be described as a mountain riddled with deep gorges, giant boulders, and dense forests that must be climbed in order to reach the sunny peak of high level wellness, maximum longevity, and enhanced quality of life. The obstacles start with the recognition of negative lifestyles, and go on to include action to reduce them, elimination of risk factors, and adoption of positive lifestyles. This leads to optimum physical, mental, and social functioning. In contrast, instead of ascending, one can take the easier trail and descend into the valley of illness and death. Many people are speeded along this descent by negative lifestyles, symptoms, signs, disease, and disability; at the bottom they fall into premature death.

A complement to Wellness is Health Promotion. It is the *process* of creating awareness of health risks, influencing attitudes and identifying alternatives. The goal is to motivate people to improve their health and environment in order that they may function at their optimum level. Wellness means fostering attitudes and actions which can lead to health and ultimately, to reduce health care costs for both employer and employee.[3]

Given this state of confusion in the interpretations of wellness, I first want to provide a context for a more indepth examination of wellness and the wellness movement. The wellness movement is representative of some very significant changes occurring in our society. By seeing wellness within this larger cultural context, we can better grasp the meaning of these changes and comprehend their significance and the possibilities that may exist for the occupational therapy profession in the domain of wellness.

Context, as defined in Webster's dictionary, is "the whole situation, background, or environment relevant to some happening . . ." It also means to "weave together"—as "the parts of a sentence, paragraph, or discourse that occur just before and after a specified word or passage and determine its exact meaning, as it is unfair to quote this remark out of its *context*".

A way of visualizing context is to think of a bowl of salad. The bowl provides the context for its contents, which may include tomatoes, lettuce, onions, and whatever else one puts in salad. In business there are frequent references to the "big picture" which is the context for many specific business activities and decisions. Because context provides a sense of the whole situation, background, or environment relevant to some happening I want to present some thoughts about a shift in cultural changes so that you will have a cultural context for my further discussion of wellness.

CULTURAL CHANGES AND WELLNESS

These thoughts originated in a book entitled, *New Rules*, by Daniel Yankelovich. Yankelovich goes beyond observed trends like those in *Megatrends* to look at (1) the cultural, or shared meanings of trends and (2) the psychological, or inner and private meaning of trends.[4]

Yankelovich proposes that out of the American search for self-fulfillment there apparently is emerging a genuine cultural revolution, or a revolution in shared meanings. He uses two principles of Hannah Arendt's work to define cultural revolutions.

Arendt's first principle is that a true revolution always begins a "new story" in human affairs: "The course of human history suddenly begins anew, an entirely new story—a story never known or told before—is about to unfold." Arendt uses the word "story" with great care and implies that the "story" of revolution will have "an inner coherence: a beginning, a middle and end, a plot line, and a meaning." This story is not mere change, for in Arendt's words, change may become a "Revolutionary shift *if* and *only if* the novelty it creates so deeply disturbs the status quo that all the old beliefs, values, meanings, traditions and structures are disturbed and profoundly modified."[4]

The shift Arendt describes is similar to shifts in perceptions brought about by transformation, paradigm shifts, and experiences with death. In some of these shifts new knowledge has been introduced, but the additive results of this knowledge do not produce the shift, nor can these shifts be brought about by intention, by planning, by intervention, or by action. Rather, as the shift occurs one's perceptions and interpretations are significantly altered, thereby producing a reorganization of values, beliefs, traditions, and thought structure.

Arendt's second principle "is that a genuine revolution will always advance the cause of human freedom" which she carefully distinguishes from liberation. Liberation is usually a product of political revolution, and it is concerned with restoring lost or abused rights. In this regard it is essentially negative: liberation from. Liberation is a right, and it can be demanded, legislated, or granted by political processes. Freedom, on the other hand, is what people do with their liberation once it is available to them. Freedom flourishes only when it involves the larger community, or what we call society or culture. In Arendt's terms, freedom occurs when citizens, in some profound sense, participate in shaping the course of their society. Freedom is elusive, and often, we know that we had it only when it is no longer available.

Within the context of these two principles, (1) the beginning of a new story in human affairs involving modification of old values, beliefs, traditions, etc., and (2) the advancement of human freedom, the founding of Colonial America was a true cultural revolution. It was revolutionary in that "Men began to doubt that poverty is inherent in the human condition. . . . The conviction that life on earth might be blessed with abundance instead of being cursed by scarcity was pre-revolutionary and American in origin; it grew directly out of the colonial experience . . ."[4]

According to Yankelovich, the founding of America met Arendt's two criteria of genuine revolution: it started a new story, beginning with the Puritans' covenant of equality before God and moved on to the translation of abstract rights into a secular society based on political freedom. It established a new chapter of human freedom as the shared meanings of America set themselves against the traditions of European heritage. The revolution was cultural rather than political, in that it revolved around shared meanings and did not result in toppled governments. The shared meaning was that mass poverty can be overcome by free people. When this was combined with other meanings, the themes of political freedom and material well-being emerged, and they have been the basis of the American dream for some two centuries.

What held these shared meanings together was the belief that a way of life built around self-denial and economic growth "paid off" for both the individual and for the country, thereby allowing private and public goals to be aligned. This growth was made possible by a hard-working, well-educated, stable, highly motivated, and product-hungry population. The "glue" that held this together was the belief in self-denial and the belief that one could succeed if one worked hard and saved. The values of acquisition and materialism maintained a strong economy. There also was a clear cut division of labor in the workplace, in homes, and in schools. In essence there was a "giving/getting contract" that worked for individuals and society.

About the turn of this century, and beginning with Taylor's scientific management (or time studies), instrumentalism, or the subordination of workers to machines, came into being. As this practice expanded in industry, we ignored the price we were paying for our industrialization: increasing numbers of giant instititutions with the accompanying depersonalizing, "objectifying," and alienating tendencies of industrial life. What we lost were the small, human-sized institutions such as local churches, neighborhoods, small schools, and family relationships that provide a sense of community and sense of self, or "the freedom to choose one's life according to one's own design".[4]

Yankelovich acknowledges the difficulty in defining community, but notes that it evokes in people the feeling that "Here is where I belong, these are my people, I care for them, they care for me, I am part of them, I know what they expect from me and I from them, they share my concerns, I know this place, I am on familiar ground, I am at home."[4]

> This is a powerful emotion, and its absence is experienced as an aching loss, a void, a sense of homelessness. The symptoms of its absence are feelings of isolation, falseness, instability, and impoverishment of spirit.

After World War II and the emergence of Maslow's writings and the Humanistic Psychology Movement, Americans engaged in a quest for self-fulfillment. In this process we concluded that the old contract, based on self-denial and hard work, should be redesigned because it failed to accommodate the existence of sacred/expressive yearnings that people discovered in the search for self-fulfillment.

According to Yankelovich what is emerging now seems to be a cultural revolution based on a new shared meaning: the assumption that it is wrong to subordinate the sacred/expressive side of man's nature to instrumentalism. What we have created is an unbalanced civilization: one in which subordination to the assembly line, to affluence, and to "me-too" has led to "insufficient concern for the values of community, expressiveness, caring, and with the domain of the sacred."[4]

The old shared meaning that marked America's first cultural revolution said that poverty was not man's destiny. The emerging, or emergent meaning says that instrumentalism is not man's destiny.

> The old meaning insisted that political freedom can exist with material well-being and indeed enhance it. The new meaning insists that the personal freedom to shape one's life can coexist with the instrumentalism of modern technological society and can civilize it.[4]

Simplistically summarized, Yankelovich states that we are on the verge of discarding Maslow's theories of self-fulfillment, which have two major flaws: "the idea of self as an aggregate of inner needs and the concept of a hierarchy of being that makes economic security a precondition to satisfying the human spirit."[4] He proposed that these theories about the self have kept us from developing a sound social ethic to replace our eroding ethic of self-denial, which brought us to the point of loss of community and self. Basically these theories brought us to a dead end. Self-fulfillment occurs when we are engaged in pursuit of a common goal with others, not when we pursue a goal in isolation.

Yankelovich predicts that an ethic of commitment is emerging now, reflecting a shift away from the self (both in self-denial and in self-fulfillment) and toward connectedness with the world.

> This commitment may be to people, institutions, objects, beliefs, ideas, places, nature, projects, experiences, adventures, and callings. It discards the Maslowian checklist of inner needs and potentials of the self, and seeks instead the elusive freedom Arendt describes as the treasure people sometimes discover when they are free to join with others in shaping the tasks and shared meanings of their times.[4]

This embryonic ethic is gathering force around two types of commitments: one is closer and deeper personal relationships and the second is a switch from certain instrumental values to sacred/expressive ones. An example of a sacred/expressive value is reverence for all living things (people, plants, wilderness, animals). Another example of sacred/expressive value is the ideal of community as reflected in the hospice movement, which rejects the instrumental efficiency of hospitals for simplicity and dignity in a community in which death is accepted as a part of life, rather than as a failure of technology.

MEANING OF CHANGES TO INDIVIDUALS

During the past year in talking and working with patients certain impressions have emerged.* Many convey the feeling

---

*It is acknowledged that the numbers of patients have been relatively small and the time period short; consequently the report of findings may be biased and should be considered as tentative.

that they search for something that is missing from their lives, the loss of which seems to be associated with feelings of loneliness and alienation, lack of peace, and a variety of symptoms—some diagnosed, some not.

Some patients have had multiple, major medical problems (such as hypertension, ulcers, diabetes, and gastro-intestinal disorders), which have interrupted their lives and often been financially devastating. They are beginning to realize that something in the way they are living may be the source, or link, among these various problems. This group includes persons who have been medically retired and are now struggling to find respect, dignity, and a place for themselves in society and their family structure.

Some patients are professionals—doctors, lawyers, managers, graduate students—all active in their professional and personal lives. Others are "well" retired persons who are diligently involved in remaining active and independent. A few people have been concerned about their health and wanted information about nutrition or exercise or lifestyle.

COMMONALITIES

What is striking is that many of these individuals seem to share some commonalities:

1. The first commonality is their *inability to be expressive* about meaningful things in their lives, especially their fears, their loss of dignity and self-worth, and the impact that role change has had for them. They have kept up with technology and information at the cost of their emotional development and dreams—both of which are basic sources of internal strength for our lives.

The histories of several medically retired patients I have seen recently suggest that they were lonely children who have become lonely adults. Even though they now have families of their own, they feel a great loss of self in the loss of their jobs. Their roles and positions in their families have changed, and frequently their wives have had to go to work, which produces further loss of self-esteem, increased anger and exacerbation of their symptoms. In some cases they are prohibited, by the terms of their retirement, from working for themselves or for anyone else.

Mini-Case #1

Arnold, at age 55, complained to me of severe pain, sadness, anger, depression and uncontrollable spells of crying because the woman with whom he had been going for two years left him. "I just can't go on like this," he said. He had been in therapy with no results; his 20 year old son who lived with him was abusing him, the insurance company was spying on him, he could not live on his retirement, and if he worked his retirement pay was reduced.

His history evolved over several sessions: "I don't ever remember anybody wanting me or defending me. My mother spent most of my childhood having nervous breakdowns or in hospitals; my father couldn't be bothered with me; my older brother beat me and humiliated me at school; I left home as soon as I could and joined the Army which was OK but the officers were always after me. I got married, had two sons, and got fired from every job I had. My wife divorced me, my older son lives with her and is going to college and doesn't have anything to do with me. I've gone with lots of women—and they all leave me. I entice them to come back—and when they do, I kick them out! Then my back goes out on me."

He had absolutely *no* awareness of any of his assets—his ability to survive, his perceptiveness, his intellect or his articulateness, among other things. This week he said, "I've lived my entire life in my mind—always reliving the past and trying to fix it. I'm scared to death to experience living in the present and to relate to people. I'm a master at failing. You know," he said, "I'm really disabled. I'm a grown man—and emotionally, I'm a scared child, and I don't know how to change that."

2. The second commonality relates to *difficulties in resolving relationship issues* with others in new situations; these patients adapt, not in a healthy, supportive way but at great cost to their health and happiness.

Mini-Case #2

I have been working with a group of senior citizens in their 70's and 80's in a stress class in which their shared experience of growing old had been a very moving and profound experience. Many of them have told of moving to Denver, or changing their living arrangements because they felt a need to be closer to their children—or they had even older relatives who came to live with them. They gave up emotional supports and friends because they needed physical help to maintain their independence. One woman described her role dilemma with the anguished question—"Am I now a parent or a child?" Fear and the consequences of alienating, or imposing upon, their children compounds this dilemma, as illustrated in this story. "My younger sister called me today and when I misunderstood her, she said 'I don't know what we're going to do with you—you always get so confused.' Well, I know my hearing is bad. I tried hearing aids once, but the noise was *so* painful. I guess I'll have to try again—but if it doesn't work, I'm afraid she'll think I'm too confused to live alone—and I'll be put away."

At that instant I knew why they had persisted throughout the course in seeking peace and harmony at the expense of their integrity. The perceived option is being sent to a nursing home.

3. A third commonality is a *desire to avoid physicians,* hospitals, and medication, particularly if the medication has any emotional or physiological side effects.

Mini-Case #3

Recently, I was trying on clothes in a small dress shop. When the clerk found out what I do, she asked to introduce me to the owner of the shop, who has a 30 year old chronic schizophrenic son. He had been fairly well controlled by medication until he learned that the medication sometimes resulted in tardive dyskinesia. Now he refuses to take his medication, presents serious behavior problems, and the family has been unable to find satisfactory and financially reasonable placement for him. In this instance, the family and the son were in need of considerable support as a result of the son's rejection of his medical treatment.

As another example of the trend away from organized medicine, The *Wall Street Journal* reported recently that Polish citizens are abandoning the state run medical care system and are turning to faith healers and others who have spiritual and sacred interests but little, if any, formal medical training. The government is obviously concerned with this trend.

4. The fourth area of commonality includes *feelings of loneliness, isolation,* and sometimes alienation among patients who have few close friends, even though they have many acquaintances and are professionally active.

Mini-Case #4

One patient was recently referred by his physician for help in controlling hypertension. He describes his situation as follows: "I am a district manager for a large, national company that is experiencing financial problems. I've been with the company 17 years, have moved my family around as required by my job, and have been in Denver about 4 years. With increasing frequency I have had to fire my employees because of the company's financial problems. This is really bothering me. I can't help them in any way, and there is no one in the company to talk with about my conflicts as the company expects that I will 'handle the job'. I have not discussed this with my wife because my own job may be threatened in a year or two, and I do not want to worry her prematurely. I've not made any friends since moving here, except for one friendship with a racketball companion, and I terminated that when he began pressing me for information about the company." He paused, tears welled up in his eyes, and he continued: "I feel really badly about being here. I've always been proud of my ability to handle my life, you know—to be macho—now I can't even do that—and I've come to a woman for help!"

5. The fifth commonality that I have observed is that in almost every instance the people I have seen and described have *medical problems and symptoms.* In some instances, the

consequences of their medical problems are as serious and disruptive for their lives and well-being as a severe physical or emotional disability can be. The major difference is that the impact of illness and disruption of life and living among this particular population of people has not been addressed. With the exception of persons who have been medically retired, most of these individuals are continuing to work and to maintain their relationships. However, they struggle mightily and expend enormous amounts of energy in their attempts to adapt and cope with the situations in their lives and in their search to find peace, meaning, or satisfaction. If this energy was available for creative and constructive pursuits, I have no doubt but that their contributions to society would be significant.

6. The sixth and final commonality that I have observed is *loss of creativity.*

A surgeon with whom I have been working remarked one day that the thing which was most difficult for him was his loss of creativity. He commented that he used to be extremely creative, and good, in creating and designing new surgical procedures, and now, to even think of being creative in that way seemed like another burden to add to those which are already so overwhelming.

WELLNESS REDEFINED

Based on experiences like those described above, I must describe wellness in a way that differs from earlier descriptions in this paper.

Wellness provides, in my experience, an opportunity for people to seek assistance with their problems of living, of adapting, and of coping without having a diagnostic label. It also provides an opportunity to seek help in an environment in which they see themselves as whole and complete people who also have problems. I thus define *wellness* as *a context for living.* As such, it consists of several elements. The first element is the *capacity for expressiveness,* or the ability to communicate through the barriers that tend to create loneliness and isolation. The second element is the development of a *sense of connectedness* with and commitment to others that reflects mutual care, concern, and respect. The third element is *recognition of that which is sacred,* which may include those things for which one has reverence as well as one's commitment to a job, to one's self, to others, and to one's community. The fourth element is that of *creating roles* that are *important in all phases of one's life.* The fifth element is *care of one's body,* through the adoption and practice of physical fitness, good nutrition, stress management, adequate rest, and environmental sensitivity. Finally, there is an element of *mastery in handling breakdowns*—an ability to flow with the ups and downs of life, keeping them in relative balance without being overwhelmed.

As people move toward a wellness lifestyle a sacred or spiritual caring for oneself develops and is reflected in the healing of old wounds and the creation of relationships that are constructive and supportive rather than reactive and destructive. The use of one's creative processes to contribute to the betterment of mankind emerges. Caring for one's body assumes more importance because there is recognition that our bodies are the vessels for our minds, emotions, and spirits. Our bodies are the vehicles through which we interact with others.

The myth of wellness is that it is a "thing" which one can "get," or an object that we can mold. In reality, it is a way of living, a state of being, a place to come from as we go about our lives. It offers untold new possibilities for us and will be reflected in our relations with others.

In the earlier interpretations of wellness, wellness seemed to be viewed as a thing, or an object, which, if people had, would produce some "other result." Frequently that "other result" was lowered insurance payments, increased profits, or better nutrition or physical fitness. Within the context of these interpretations, wellness becomes merely another form of our eroding ethic of instrumentalism—a subordination of people to a product, a process, or a process that produces a product.

The reality of wellness, and the possibilities inherent in wellness, when viewed from the perspective of Yankelovich's theory that an ethic of commitment is emerging, are many. Wellness, as a context for living, is a state of being, a place to come from as we commit ourselves to improving life for all of us. As a context for living, wellness is not limited to getting something for me—rather it becomes the possibility that my life, my wellness, contributes to you and to your wellness. It thus is available to all—regardless of whether we are healthy or terminally ill.

Mini-Case #5

Recently I was working with a physician who was seeing me for his stress-related problems. He has his own hospital, a new family, and two children from a previous marriage who live with him. He prides himself on being a strict disciplinarian, a perfectionist, and as one who has exacting standards for himself and for others. He has been very successful, but the price he has paid in terms of his own sense of well-being and peace has been enormous. Even he had begun to be worried about his outbursts of anger and his ways of dealing with people who do not perform according to his standards. One day he described to me two instances in which he dealt with his two older children. In the first instance, he responded very angrily to the older child's behavior, and he thought his anger was appropriate to the situation. In the second instance, the younger child stated a desire to purchase some equipment for a pet, for which a considerable amount of money had been spent earlier in the summer. His response was "No, you've spent too much money on that animal already." The child then said, "But I earned it, and I don't see why I can't spend it if I want to." He acknowledged her point and then said, "Tell me the reasons that you think this is important, and if you can convince me that your argument is logical, I will support you." The child then presented some very appropriate arguments.

My client supported her thinking, and then he described what he had told and demonstrated to her about ways in which she could be very effective in dealing with other people. When he finished I ask him if he realized what a powerful and effective role model he had been in that situation. Initially, he did not perceive that he had done anything positive (which was not an uncommon perception for him), but it provided an excellent opportunity to bring to his awareness and to reinforce the existence of a variety of resources and options that he had available and had not recognized or utilized. The point of this story is that it provided the opportunity and impetus for him to examine his responses to people, and he is now beginning to make some very significant modifications in his perception of himself and his relationships with others. He, like most people wants to contribute to others and will do so if given the opportunity or possibility.

POTENTIALS FOR OCCUPATIONAL THERAPY IN WELLNESS SERVICES

Given the perspective of wellness as a context for living, what are the possibilities for occupational therapy practice in the domain of wellness? Specifically, what are the possibilities for *private practice* in the domain of wellness? I believe that there are significant possibilities, and the most important opportunity exists in patient, or client, populations with whom we have done little in recent years.

For Those With Stress Related Symptoms

For lack of better descriptors at this time, individuals with stress-related symptoms are excellent candidates for us and the service we have the potential to make available. These individuals are truly suffering—physically, emotionally, and in terms of their relationships with others. My experience so far, which is limited, suggests that people who suffer from stress—or who struggle with it—have highly developed cognitive resources, but their emotional maturity and self-esteem are poorly developed. Consequently, attempts to adapt and to cope with the demands of their lives require inordinate amounts of energy. Occupational therapy, if perceived as an interactive laboratory for experience, for action, for socialization, and for communications, can make very significant contributions to emotional development and building of self-esteem.

There is an adage about learning that says:

I hear—I forget
I see—I remember
I act—I understand and change.

To see, to hear, to think are all internal processes. To act produced a result: feedback is a consequence of action and it stimulates learning and change. The quotation in our profession that "we make doing possible": or Reilly's statement that, "Man, through the use of his hands, as they are energized by mind and will, influences the state of his health," attest to the power of action in bringing forth changes in our lives.

While there are few prospective studies about the ability of life-style changes to prevent illness or disease, much work is being done in this area, and I think that we can position ourselves to be forerunners in lifestyle change. When we know what questions to ask, I believe we will find evidence to support the importance of life-style change, and I think it is possible that occupational therapists could effectively do some of that research. The August 30, 1984, issue of *The New England Journal of Medicine* had a report of a prospective study conducted by the Health Insurance Plan of Greater New York. The study used a sample of over 2,000 patients who had had one heart attack. The finding was that lonely, isolated men, with less than a 10th grade education, and who hold low level jobs over which they have little control, are four times more likely to die of a second heart attack than are other individuals. The Type A theory of personality was shown to be poor predictor of death from a second heart attack.[5]

In an accompanying editorial, Dr. Thomas B. Graboys of Harvard Medical School wrote: "We can probably obtain as much information about a given patient's risk of dying by talking about what's going on in his life, as by conducting an exhaustive examination with the latest in medical technology."

For Those With Severe Medical Problems

In addition to working with persons with stress, who very frequently have numerous medical symptoms, although not always diagnosed problems, a second potential population appropriate for occupational therapists consists of persons with severe medical problems, such as hypertension, ulcers, diabetes, obesity, hernias, and gastro-intestinal conditions. These individuals are also disabled, not necessarily in the same way that persons with physical or emotional illnesses are disabled—but no less so in terms of being able to handle their lives and contribute to their own care and the care of others. Among this group are persons who have been medically retired from their jobs and who are suffering from their illnesses as well as their loss of self-esteem, pride, and dignity. Frequently these individuals are in poor physical condition, have poor nutritional habits, and experience high levels of stress. A modified version of some occupational therapy outpatient rehabilitation programs would probably do wonders for patients in this category, and might, incidentally, save significant amounts of money currently being spent for their medical care.

For Those Disillusioned With Medical Care

One other issue that, from my perspective,' offers possibilities for private practice, is the growing disillusionment with traditional medical care. A significant number of the patients that I have seen want nothing more to do with physicians or hospitals, primarily because they have experienced depersonalization and believe physicians and other health care providers do not listen to them. Many of these individuals are today spending significant amounts of their personal money with a variety of health care providers who are sensitive not only to the physical complaints but to their emotional needs: rolfers, chiropractors, astrologers, persons who give massages, and persons utilizing a variety of forms of Eastern therapies, such as Jin Shin Jyuitsui. With this particular group of people, I believe that a therapist needs to be highly ethical, particularly in terms of observing any symptoms or complaints that may be indicative of need for medical treatment and should make every effort to support such individuals in seeking qualified medical care.

OCCUPATIONAL THERAPY WELLNESS SERVICES— IMPLICATIONS

What are some of the implications for delivering services in a wellness model? The first implication is recognition of the fact that many of the people who do seek services in such a setting have problems, symptoms, or something that is of concern to them—and yet they either consider themselves to be basically well or they want to be well. In other words, they do not want to be seen as their pathology. On the other hand well persons may not necessarily come to wellness centers. When people feel well, they do not seem to be very conscious of their bodies, although they may really like the way they feel as a result of their exercise or nutritional habits. As Will Rogers said, "If it ain't broke—don't fix it!" This awareness is important in terms of marketing a "wellness" program.

The second implication for practice in a wellness program relates to the relationship with the patient and the therapist. In a "wellness" environment, there is an opportunity to work with the patient in the context of his life. This has created a shift in the way that I view the knowledge, skills, and wisdom I bring to our sessions. I see myself less as a teacher or therapist and more as a coach whose job is to bring forth the resources that the patient has and to provide an environment in which he can test and experiment with those resources, thereby acquiring mastery in their use. Sometimes this requires that I see strengths and resources that the patient may not see, or of which the patient is unaware. Sometimes it means that together we have to bring about a shift in a self-perceptions and a shift in views of using resources. It often means dealing with the unknown. More specifically, I may know nothing about the problem area with which we are working, but I do know that I have knowledge and skills that enable the patient to become masterful in handling those issues.

The third implication is that working in the area of wellness puts the occupational therapist right into the community in which the patient lives, plays, and works. Consequently, the agenda items which have priority are the patient's rather than the therapist's or the institution's. Since the patient may be paying the bill, he must be intimately involved in identifying the issues to be addressed and committed to developing strategies for resolving those issues. This requires a very direct relationship between the therapist and patient, one based on mutual respect for each other and the resources that each brings. The patient's problems can be viewed as breakdowns in areas in which the patient needs to acquire mastery and the possibility exists that the patient has the resources to become masterful but does not recognize those resources or know how to use them. In other words, self-healing is a basic part of the process.

The fourth implication for practice is that the people who seek services are most often people who want assistance in dealing with something that is missing in their lives. They do not want to be viewed as being "sick" or as having a pathological problem. They want to be in an environment in which they experience being treated and seen as a complete person, not as a pathological condition.

The final implication of which I am currently aware is that as we work with patients in the domain of wellness, particularly when wellness is viewed as a context for living, the questions that we ask will be significantly different than the questions we ask in more traditional medical settings. For example, given the use of diagnostic related groups and other pressures that limit treatment costs, in medical settings, the questions asked relate to the pathological condition. What is wrong, and what does the patient need to have to be self-sufficient? We then refer to the "menial" but important tasks of feeding and dressing oneself.

In a wellness environment, the question becomes: What does this patient want to do with his life and how can we together make that possible? How do we transform possibility into action? How often I have heard that we must make sure our patients have realistic goals when, in fact our jobs are to support the client in bringing forth whatever possibilities exist for him—instead of imposing limits.

CONCLUSION

The gem in this learning experience is that we, as human beings, are limited only by what we think is possible. If we open ourselves to new possibilities, our world expands enormously. We have only to remember what Yankelovich identified as the true cultural revolution that came out of America's founding: the recognition that poverty is not destiny—and the emerging recognition that man does not have to be subordinated to machines.

Similarly, our jobs are to bring forth possibilities for our patients and clients—and to work with them on the steps that turn possibility into reality. When viewed from this perspective, feeding and dressing are no longer menial tasks—they are basic steps on the way to some greater possibility, and we need never apologize for having that as a part of our responsibility.

The challenge to practice in the area of wellness may be (1) reimbursement, for I do not know to what extent insurance companies will pay for what I have described and (2) the need for education at the graduate level. Within the possible constraints of these two challenges, I believe that private practice offers limitless possibilities.

In conclusion, a patient of mine who is a public relations specialist described an incident with one of her clients. "We were down to the wire on a printing job which had a close deadline for a workshop. In reading the final proofs, my client decided he wanted to make changes to more accurately reflect his business philosophy. I explained the risks and deadlines to him, and he conceded that it was not possible to make the changes. When I got home, I said to myself: 'Am I in the business of telling people what their limits are—or am I in the business of creating possibilities?' "

As occupational therapists, we must individually ask ourselves that very same question.

I have no hesitancy in saying that we are in the business of creating possibilities for and with our patients. I make that commitment with the knowledge that we can create the environment and provide the support and guidance that produce results out of those possibilities. The risks are numerous, and yet I believe our commitment to our patients will provide us with the strength and courage to prevail, even when the health care system insists on cost containment and efficiency.

My optimism about the potential for our profession has never been higher. I invite you to join me in fulfilling the challenge of bringing forth the dreams that our patients have for their lives and to join our patients in bringing their dreams to fruition.

REFERENCES

1. —————. Establishing priorities in the wellness program, *Occup Health and Safety* 35: June 1982

2. Morefield J: Runaway employee health care costs: Remedies for the Future, *Time Magazine*, Special Advertising Section June 18, 1984

3. Berry CA, Berry MA: Wellness: A positive strategy for a healthy business, *Time Magazine*, Special Advertising Section June 18, 1984

4. Yankelovich D: *New Rules*. New York: Bantam Books 1981

5. Ruberman WM, Weinblat E, Goldberg JD, Chaudhary BS: Psychosocial influences on mortality after myocardial infarction, *NE Jo Med* 331:552–559 Aug 30 1984

6. Graboys TB: Stress and the aching heart, *NE Jo Med* 311:594–595 Aug 30 1984